THE ACUPRESSURE WARMUP

for Fitness, Athletic Preparation and Injury Management

MARC COSEO

Paradigm Publications, Brookline, Massachusetts 1992

The Acupressure Warm-up
by Marc Coseo
© 1992 Paradigm Publications

Library of Congress Cataloging–in–Publication Data
Coseo, Marc, 1958–
   The acupressure warmup: a system of athletic preparation and injury prevention/
Marc Coseo.
       p.   cm.
   Includes bibliographical references and index.
   ISBN 0-912111-34-8 : $16.95
   1.Acupressure. 2.Sports — Accidents and injuries — Prevention.
3.Physical fitness. I.Title.
RM723.A27C67   1992
615.8'22--dc20   92–419
                                        CIP

Published in the United States by
Paradigm Publications, Brookline, MA

Distributed in the U.S.A.
  to the book trade by Talman & Co, New York
  and to the health professions by Redwing Book Co, Brookline, MA

Distributed in the EEC by CYGNUS Buchimport, Munich

Cover design by Jack Boyce
Typesetting and graphics by EPS, Boston, MA 02129

0987654321

TABLE OF CONTENTS

THE ADDED EDGE

WHEN WE BEGIN an athletic endeavour, we face a mountain of difficulty; not only physical, but also intellectual and emotional challenge. It is our personal mountain, one we must ascend by ourselves. As we climb, we find new sources of self-confidence, a seemingly endless supply of energy, extraordinary dedication and devotion. In this sense, but in a far more positive light, athletics is like the labors of Sisyphus, the legendary king of Corinth who was condemned to roll a boulder up a mountain forever, only to have it roll down again once he reached the top. Of course, unlike Sisyphus, we impose athletic labors on ourselves. Having once felt the confidence, energy and dedication climbing the mountain brings, we develop a positive hunger that goes hand in hand with success. In short, we choose to climb our own mountain forever.

In athletics, struggle is personal; each mountain is made of individual limitations, goals, and priorities. However, there always comes a time when we must push harder than is comfortable. This is what makes an athlete grow. The more effort we expend, the greater our personal reward. To ascend our personal mountain, we must put ourselves on the line again and again if we are to reach our goal. It is then that physical injury is most likely to take its toll and that the Acupressure Warmup will help you most.

The Acupressure Warmup is based on the same practical theories that helped acupuncture climb the medical mountain. It has survived 2,000 years as a medical system, while modern medicine has existed less than a century. But, the survival of acupuncture was neither luck, nor magic; it survived because it is practical. Simply stated, it worked for so many people that it was never lost.

As you learn and use the Acupressure Warmup you will see that it is practical too. It's fast, safe, simple, and extremely effective at loosening those tight muscles that stretching cannot touch. You will find yourself more keenly aware of what your body tells you. You will know your body, its limitations, its potentials, and how to give it a proper chance to fit your athletic dreams and ambitions.

PREFACE

I WAS IN college training for tennis six hours a day, seven days a week. The rest of the time I attended classes and studied. I was into it. I was going somewhere and nothing could possibly stop me. A day off tennis was hell; two days off wasn't imaginable. I felt so strongly about the game and was so driven to succeed that any injury was devastating. But, because I trained so long and hard, injuries were a common occurrence. Most of my injuries were minor. Once I broke my foot and once I cracked my wrist. Otherwise, my impairments were the tennis player's standards — back spasms, sprained ankles, twisted knees, pulled stomach muscles.

Once, ten days after pulling a muscle in my back, I was moping around my apartment in a manner unique to an injured athlete. To take my mind off my woes my roommate Curt persuaded me to go to the mall and play video games. That lasted about five minutes. I decided to walk to a bookstore and look for a book on sports injuries. Once there I asked the store manager where I could find such a book. She said she didn't know of any off-hand but, if they existed, they would be in the fifth or sixth aisle. I went where she directed, looked down, and saw a book on prescription medicine. Wrong aisle. In the next aisle I came to a section on massage and skimmed through the books. I found one about this chinesey stuff called "acupressure."

I picked up the book, skimmed it, stopped and read a bit, skimmed it some more. Then, I discovered a diagram with a round dot exactly where my back hurt. "Hmmmm," I thought, "this looks interesting." I bought the book, left the store feeling hopeful, returned to the video arcade, retrieved my roommate, went home and read the book.

Most of the points it recommended to "ease back spasms" were in places that I could neither reach nor push hard enough to achieve the "desired stimulus." Being of sound mind and mightily tired of my mopey mood, my roommate agreed to help apply pressure to points the book recommended. When we finished my first-ever acupressure treatment, I told Curt that I seemed to feel a little better. Curt looked at me and said, "Feel better! Man, you're standing straight." He was right; it was the first time in ten days that I had straightened my back. We looked at each other and almost simultaneously said, "Hey! this stuff works!"

About forty minutes later my back began to hurt again but less than before. I was also getting a little bent over again. I asked Curt to do the same acupressure points again, and got the same positive results. Forty minutes passed, an hour went by, then I felt a slight twinge. An hour and a half passed before I started to bend over again. Each time Curt applied acupressure, the effects would last longer. Eventually, Curt got tired of being an "acupressurist" and went to his room to read.

Later that afternoon, I noticed a mother, her son, and his dog playing in the park. His dog was a collie, he was a curtain crawler. His mother gave him the ball and he'd throw it about five feet. Occasionally, because his mother could see how frustrated the dog was, she'd throw the ball. The collie would be back in thirty seconds wagging its tail. The boy was laughing and clapping, the dog was running around, and even the look on the mother's face as she wiped saliva from her hands inspired memories of dog-ball with my own labrador retriever.

I remembered throwing the ball as far as I could; she'd bring it back, wet of course, and I'd throw it again. Once in a while she'd play keep away and I'd pretend to throw the ball but hide it behind my back, standard stuff for a boy and his dog. That day though, I remembered a part of the scene I'd forgotten. My labrador would wedge an old tennis ball between her back and the ground, then roll on it. With her eyes half closed and a chorus of pleasant grunts it was obvious that she was enjoying herself. After a minute or so she would get up, stretch, shake the grass off her coat and, in hind-sight, look at me to say "What, Marc, you've never heard of acupressure?"

Tennis Balls! Of course!

Lying on tennis balls turned out to be better than Curt's treatments. Not only was I able to control the pressure but I could spend all the time I needed to get my back to relax. When I finished, I could hardly contain myself. I pounded on my roommate's door and told him about it. Of course, he was pleased. He must have been saying to himself, "This is great, I won't have to do that anymore." I used the tennis ball tech-nique one more time and then went to bed happy that I'd soon be playing tennis again.

When I woke up the next morning, I found that my back had tightened a little dur-ing the night. Breakfast became second on my list of things to do. I grabbed the balls from the kitchen table and started in on my new routine. I repeated the process three more times that day even though my back didn't hurt after the second try. The follow-ing day I was hitting against a wall and a day later I was playing a match.

From then on, whenever I had a muscle injury I would use the same technique. Sometimes, when the points were easy to reach, I would apply the pressure with just my thumbs or fingers. Seeing how useful it was for treating injuries, I began using it as a warmup. By the time I was playing the pro tour I was using an eight point warmup rou-tine every day. Despite my even more trying schedule, my injury rate stayed low. My respect for acupressure's power made me increasingly interested in the Oriental philoso-phies and medicine from which it grew. I often asked myself, "If this works so well and has been around for 2,000 years, why don't more people here use it?"

When you depend on your body for a living, you learn quickly that you cannot spend a lot of time injured. Thus the Oriental idea of prevention came to mean a lot to me. In ancient times Oriental doctors didn't get paid unless their patients remained healthy. It was believed that a good practitioner could treat an imbalance before it became an injury or a disease. By recognizing imbalance before it was too late, doctors kept their patients healthy.

Of course, the Warmup evolved into a preventative system not only because I was impressed by the Oriental philosophy of health but also because my injury rate had improved so dramatically. I typically used it twice a day, once when I got up and once when I went to bed. In the world of athletics, people are more in tune with their bodies and more open to new ideas. So, it was probably inevitable that it would evolve further, becoming a system that I could teach to others.

Once, in Le Tourquet, France, the morning before my third round match, I decided to do the Acupressure Warmup in the player's lounge. No one was around and, if they were, lying on tennis balls wouldn't be the strangest thing a player did on tour. So I was taking my time, letting the acupressure relax my muscles. Fifteen minutes later I opened my eyes to see a woman staring at me from across the room. She said, *"Excusez-moi monsieur Coseo, j'aimerais savoir ce que vous etes en train de faire."* I did what my dog would have done, not understanding a single word. I got up, brushed the lint from my warmup, stretched and said, "Haven't you heard of acupressure before?" She said, *"Non."* I said, "You will!" I taught her after my match. I couldn't speak French and she couldn't speak English but apparently she learned. The next day I saw her teaching it to some of her friends.

While in Portugal playing a tournament, I had a right of way dispute with a car. I was a pedestrian, the car was a Renault. It won. I took a long time to recover. This time I didn't even try video games to deal with my frustration.

I applied to the New England School of Acupuncture, which had a reputation for being the best in the U.S. During my education I began to understand why acupressure worked and learned how clinical experts applied the acupuncture points. I researched how the routine I had begun as an injured athlete could be developed to help others.

After graduation, I opened an acupuncture practice and began treating patients for sports injuries. Between treatments I would have them do "homework." Homework was those portions of the Acupressure Warmup most applicable to their injury. Invariably they came back to rave about how much better they felt after applying acupressure the first time. Most of my patients continue to use the Acupressure Warmup to prevent further injury.

Today, I offer you this system with my hope that it will help you stay injury free, and keep you in hot pursuit of your athletic ambitions.

INTRODUCTION

WHY USE THE
ACUPRESSURE WARMUP?

Up UNTIL A YEAR AGO no one questioned stretching as a warmup prior to competition or working out. Although stretching was an advance over calisthenics, which had been the only warmup for many years, using stretching as a preparatory routine has done little to lessen injuries in sports. In fact, more sports injuries occur today than ever before. James Garrick, the Director of the Center for Sports Medicine at Saint Francis Hospital, believes that one of the main causes of sports injuries today is improper stretching. In the March 5th, 1990 issue of *U.S. News and World Report*, Dr. Garrick states, "We see more injuries in people trying to get flexible than those that are tight to start with."

If we strive for flexibility when our muscles are still inelastic and cold we are forcing them to do something that they can't yet do. Their response is a mechanism called the stretch reflex. When our muscles are forced to stretch beyond normal limits, sensory impulses travel from the muscle tissue to the spinal cord. After the brain receives and interprets the data, a signal returns to the muscle instructing it to contract. This natural, protective contraction is then opposed by the attempt to stretch, causing a muscular tug-of-war between your muscles' self-defense and your desire to become more flexible. This leads to muscle tears, which lead to scar tissue and diminished flexibility. In addition, your tendons become inflamed and your ligaments tend to loosen. This eventually leads to joint instability.

In short, stretching doesn't solve the preparation problem and may even make things worse. When we force our bodies to bend and flex beyond their limits, we damage ligaments and tissues that are essential to movement. When the stress of exercise demands more oxygen and nutrients than are available, or when our circulation is inadequate to carry away the waste products of a stressed metabolism, cramps and stiffness are a common result. Tight muscles and poor circulation reduce flexibility and contribute to breaks and tears. Repeated damage can lead to pain, reduced range of movement and, in some cases, to problems requiring surgery.

To understand how the Acupressure Warmup solves these problems, think about why we call it "warming up." When things get warm, they become looser and more flexible. Solids are less brittle and bend more easily, liquids flow more smoothly, and tight spots expand. Our muscles exhibit the same characteristics. When they are warm they are less likely to become injured and are more responsive to our athletic demands. In short, our muscles exhibit flexibility in direct proportion to increased temperature.

The Acupressure Warmup provides a way to increase muscle temperature without force or strain. It consists of twenty two acupoints that affect groups of tendons, muscles and ligaments that are highly stressed in sports and fitness routines. The choice of points was determined by both clinical and personal experience in the treatment of musculoskeletal problems. Pressure at these points stimulates greater microcirculatory activity in the tissue bed, which produces a more efficient movement of blood at the capillary level. With this increased circulation of blood, the necessary heat and nutrients are delivered to muscle tissue. Because of the positive impact heat has on our muscles, we become more supple and less prone to injury.

Because acupressure offers us 2,000 years of clinical experience, we are able to use that experience to choose points that have the greatest effect on the muscle groups, tendons, ligaments, and nerves that are used in sports. Thus it provides a more systematically complete warmup than any single activity or stretching routine. Since it is easy and quick, you'll have plenty of time to do the special stretching exercises we have included. These stretches are based on the same meridian system accessed by acupressure. Since meridian stretches don't require forcing your muscles, they don't initiate the stretch reflex. Since they follow the acupressure exercises, your body will already be more supple. Performed with thoughtful concentration they can also serve as a guide to your condition.

How to use the
Acupressure Warmup

THIS BOOK has three main parts. In the first part you will learn twenty-two exercises that access the meridian system and important acupoints. Seventeen of these points are activated with tennis balls and five are activated with finger pressure. The second part of the book describes twelve stretches that are similar to the stretching exercises you may already use. However, these stretches have been developed from Oriental arts allied to acupressure — qi gong and tai chi — and help you "groove in" the benefits of the warmup. In the third section you will learn several flexibility tests you may use to keep track of your progress.

At the beginning, do each of the exercises or stretches one at a time, stopping to use the book, learning as you go. Later, when you are familiar with the exercises and stretches, all the exercises and stretches can be completed in one steady, fluid routine.

The first twenty two exercises are presented in four units:

• Information concerning the acupoint.

• Point location, always one point on each side of your body.

• Instructions for positioning your body.

• Instructions for activating the points.

From the first seventeen exercises you will learn how to place two tennis balls where they will activate an important acupoint and for five exercises you will do the same with finger pressure alone. You will also find experience notes, hints from others who use the routine. For your convenience and ease of use, each part of each exercise is always in the same place and format.

The general discussions sometimes mention diseases or conditions for which the acupoint is used by professional acupuncturists in the Orient. These applications have been included to give you a sense of the practical clinical value of the acupoints. If you recognize a problem that you or your friends or family have experienced, remember that this information is only part of the story and nothing can replace the advice of an experienced health care professional. In other words, this is a warmup book, not a list of home remedies.

Point Locations

There are several ways of locating the Acupressure Warmup points. In the introduction to each exercise there are two written descriptions, one using modern anatomical language, the other using body landmarks to describe the point location. For each point you will also find a step-by-step procedure illustrated with photographs. Follow these instructions and you will find the point. The instructions are supported by sketches showing the location and photographs illustrating the procedure.

Finding the acupoints is easy because the meridians and points are proportional to your overall size, shape, and weight. Thus, point finding is done with fingerwidths and handwidths. Most importantly, you will feel the points. The anatomical description and the point finding procedure are meant to get you close to the point. The exact location is found by touch. The point is exactly where you find the unique achy feeling associated with an acupoint. This feeling is similar to what you feel when receiving a deep massage. Generally, the achy sensation will be felt immediately; if you can't feel it, adjust your posture or move the balls slightly until you do.

For most normally healthy people the achy feeling subsides in fifteen to twenty seconds. There is a tendency for acupressure points that are related to a problem to be "reactive." That is, the achy sensation will tend to be stronger and last longer. However, everyone's sensitivity to acupoints is a little different and you should use the sensation as a guide without attempting to draw conclusions from it.

BODY POSITIONING

The postures you will learn are designed so that your body weight provides the pressure that activates the acupoints. Since your weight and size are proportional to the pressure required to activate the point, you will learn to apply appropriate pressure with very little practice. Then, you can relax and concentrate on feeling the point and the surrounding muscles. Keep in mind that the postures are guides, not drills; what counts is the acupoint activation. While the postures described are comfortable, everyone is different and you should not hesitate to modify and customize the postures for yourself.

As designed, all the exercises can be performed on any surface where you can lie down comfortably. You need no more space than is necessary to lie flat. Remember that you are warming up. Don't use any surface that makes you feel cold. Grass, artificial playing surfaces, concrete courts and gym floors are all suitable. The exercises can even be modified for use on benches and walls. The main principles are these:

Be comfortable; don't force or strain.

Be steady; increase or decrease the pressure gradually.

Be patient; listen to your body — more and faster are **not** better.

Be moderate; never cause pain. Stay warm; don't get wet or cold.

The effects will last longer than other warmup routines with which you may be familiar. You may warm up on your living room floor and still be loose and ready when you arrive on site for your game. Just as you have learned to judge other aspects of your mental and physical preparedness, you will learn to time this for yourself. By the way, the Acupressure Warmup is also a great "cool down." After an intense match or workout, when you know you will be stiff and sore, try it and see.

When the twenty-two exercises are used in sequence, you will be able to develop an easy flow from one to the next. However, as you gain awareness, learning which points are most achy and require the most attention, you can also design a personal routine by abbreviating or skipping exercises that address areas where you need less work.

All of these points can be massaged. If you feel a strain in the middle of a match, for example, firmly rub the point that you know affects the strained area. Use enough pressure to get the achy feeling, then rub it away.

ACTIVATING THE POINTS

The points are activated by pressure. This pressure is applied by positioning two tennis balls, one on each point, on each side of the body. On some points you will activate both right and left sides simultaneously — for example, all the points on the back. For points on the sides, arms and legs, the postures activate one point at a time. In all cases, follow this general procedure:

1. Find the point.
2. Get into the right posture.
3. Place the balls at the point(s).
4. Lower your weight onto the ball(s) gradually until an "achy" feeling is produced by the pressure of the ball against the point.
5. As the ache diminishes, increase the pressure by relaxing, or shifting your weight onto the balls.
6. Retain the maximum pressure you can keep without pain for as long as you can feel the ache diminishing, and the surrounding muscles relaxing.

"Ache" is not pain, but a dull sensation that diminishes over time. Everyone's response to pressure at each of the acupoints is different. In fact, your response to the same point will differ depending on your current state of health and condition. When you are using the Acupressure Warmup to get ready for an event, or as part of a daily routine, twenty to thirty seconds of pressure on each point is sufficient. At this pace the entire warmup takes about ten minutes. However, when time is short, move quickly through the routine. Even a two-minute high speed tour of the points is better than no warmup at all.

The flex-tests and stretches can be skipped, the balls can be moved quickly from point to point, and all the points can be sufficiently activated. Later, as you know your response to the points better, and have gained a deeper sensitivity to your condition, you can abbreviate your routine to save time. Simply concentrate on those points that most affect what you know you need. Return to the entire routine whenever you are not rushed.

Here are a few guidelines:

The greater the ache, the more you need to activate the point.

A fast warmup is better than no warmup at all.

Pain is a warning; never ignore pain that has no clear cause.

You will quickly learn to recognize the distinctive ache that indicates a point is active. This is a good informal gauge of condition. If the point is achy, you know that you have found the point correctly and that further activation is required. As the ache subsides, you know that activating the point has helped.

Ache is not a matter for concern; however, pain should always be carefully considered. When you experience pain and its cause is a cut, bruise, or other clearly identified injury, work around the area. Try the point closest to it with light, gradual pressure, or even just a gentle self-massage. Try to get the achy sensation. If you are experiencing pain, especially recurring pain with no clear cause, see your doctor.

CAUTIONS

These procedures are for people whose physical condition is suitable for participation in sports. If your doctor has told you that your condition is not suitable for some sports, these exercises still should pose no problem. However, you should consult with your physician first. Nothing in this book can replace or is meant to replace medical advice. If you have any question, show your doctor the book. He or she may recognize some of the flex-tests, will know your condition and may even be familiar with the benefits of acupuncture or acupressure. If your physician suggests eliminating or modifying an exercise, follow that advice.

There is no general reason why physically challenged athletes, or people with temporary physical impairments, cannot use these exercises. However, individual conditions vary and you should consult your physician if you have any concern. The following conditions are examples of situations where advice should be sought:

- Any surgery.
- Any injury, cut, break or tear.
- Any recurring pain the cause of which is not clear.
- Any disease affecting your joints.
- Any pain that always occurs when you perform a specific movement.

Complementary medical professionals, acupuncturists and Oriental massage therapists, physical therapists, chiropractors, and others can also help with specific problems.

BASIC EXERCISES

LOOKING BACK
GB–20

LOOKING BACK is so named because of its ability to relieve neck tension. If your neck is stiff, you will have trouble turning to look behind. When you wake up in the morning with a stiff neck, after sleeping in an odd position, GB-20 is the point of choice. There is another interesting observation about LOOKING BACK that you can make for yourself. When you next come down with a cold, check to see if the back of your neck feels sore. While activating GB-20 won't cure your cold, you may be surprised at how quickly this point relieves the muscular tension.

Your athletic capabilities are often controlled by your ability to perceive what is happening around you. If you are unable to turn your head smoothly and comfortably, you are handicapped by a diminished field of perception. With diminished perception, you won't receive all the information possible. Without maximal information, you won't perform to your full potential.

LOCATION
GB–20

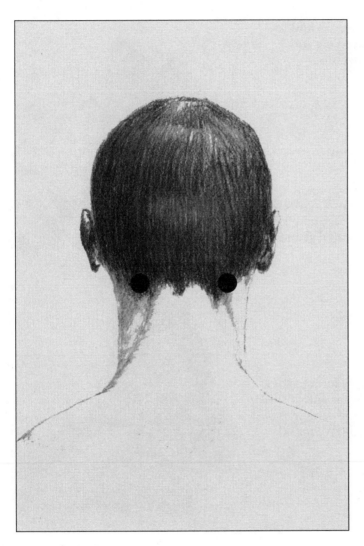

LOCATION

GB-20 is located at the back of the neck, inside the hair-line, in a depression created by the origins of the two large muscles that run down the neck.

LOCAL ANATOMY

The sternocleidomastoid and trapezius muscles begin here. Both these and the splenius capitus and semi-spinalis capitus muscles are affected when you activate LOOKING BACK.

HOW TO LOCATE

LOOKING BACK

1 Reach behind both ears and find the bony protrusions. Place your index fingers on these protrusions.

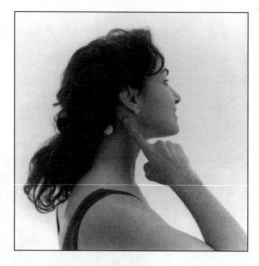

2 Slide your index finger approximately one inch toward the center of your neck until your fingers naturally fall into the depressions located at the base of your skull.

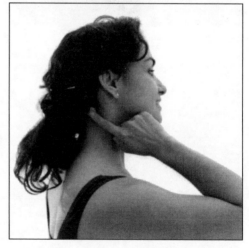

3 When your fingers have located these depressions, press upward and inward. You will feel the achy sensation that indicates you have found the points.

ACTIVATING THE POINT
GB–20

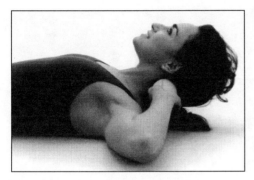

1 Lie flat, relaxed, with your feet comfortably spaced, and your neck slightly arched.

2 Place the balls in the palms of your hands and slide them beneath your neck on both sides where you found GB-20.

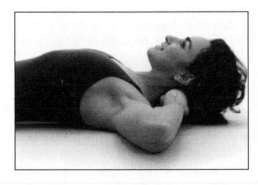

3 Lower the weight of your head and neck onto the balls. Inhale slowly and deeply so that first your abdomen, then your chest, rises with the incoming breath. Then, exhale slowly through your nose while you relax and concentrate on the feeling at the points.

EXPERIENCE NOTES

Repeat breathing deeply until the achy feeling subsides.

You may feel a sensation that goes from one or both of the points toward your ear, particularly when the points are first activated. This is a positive sign. It will generally disappear along with the ache.

The amount of weight on the balls depends on how your head touches the floor. The more you arch your neck, resting the top of your head against the floor, the less weight on the balls.

DISAPPEARING TENSION
SI-12

Virginia

Virginia was in her 60's when she first came for treatment. Although she had the vitality of someone thirty years younger, arthritis made her neck and shoulders so tense and painful that she could not turn her head from side to side. Golf had been her passion but arthritis had forced her to give it up three years earlier. Since Virginia's condition was long-standing, her therapy began with an acupuncture treatment. For two days after that treatment she applied the acupressure techniques described in this book. She concentrated on the points GB-20 (Looking Back) and SI-12 (Disappearing Tension). She applied acupressure to these points three times each day.

After the first two treatments there was a noticeable difference in her mobility. By the sixth treatment she was back on the golf course with her friends. Three years later, Virginia is still playing golf and experiences only minor flare-ups of arthritis. When she does have a flare-up, she does a little acupressure and "feels better almost immediately."

ACTIVATING THIS POINT greatly reduces tension in your neck and shoulders. The stresses and strains of modern living seem to accumulate in this area. Part of the reason for this is that our working lives so often involve sitting all day at a desk or leaning over a keyboard. Even many active jobs require keeping your head tilted forward. To accommodate this sustained posture, our bodies naturally respond by tensing the muscles in this area. As the muscles tense, circulation diminishes. As circulation diminishes, the muscles begin to lack nutrients that enable them to relax. Working constantly in this position thus becomes a vicious cycle of pain and tension. Left unattended, complications such as headaches, muscle knots and tears will begin to appear.

Because this is a point where several meridians meet, activating DISAPPEARING TENSION increases the circulation in your whole upper body. As your circulation increases, your strength and coordination will improve and you will feel loose and ready.

LOCATION
SI-12

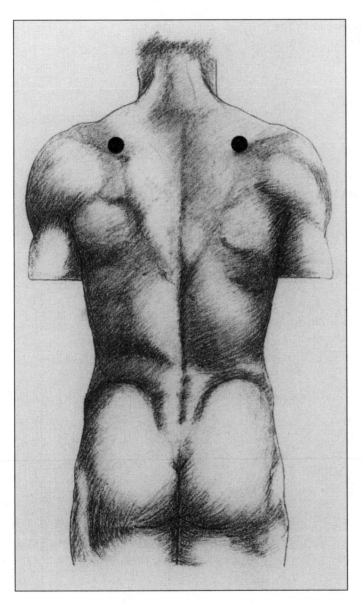

LOCATION

SI-12 is located in a depression above the bony ridge of the shoulder blade, approximately five inches from the spine.

LOCAL ANATOMY

The bony protrusion is the coracoid process of the scapula. The large muscle is the trapezius.

HOW TO LOCATE

DISAPPEARING TENSION

1 Raise your right arm outward to the side so that it is parallel to the ground with the palm of your hand facing downward.

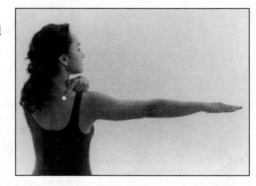

2 Reach across your body with your left hand and feel for the depression which appears when your arm is in this raised position.

NOTE: If you have trouble finding the depression, lower your arm to your side and feel for the bony ridge on top of your shoulder blade. Slide your finger upward and into the depression. Apply pressure. When you notice the achy sensation, you have found the point.

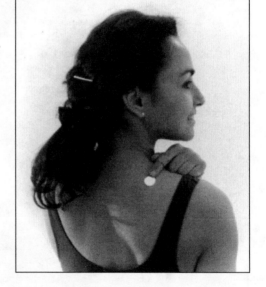

3 Repeat this process on your left side.

ACTIVATING THE POINT
SI-12

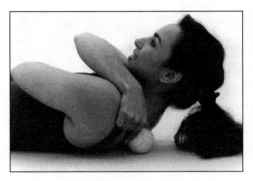

1 Begin at the end of Exercise One by removing the balls from their position at GB-20 and letting your head lie flat.

2 Elevate your left shoulder. With your right hand, place the ball under SI-12.

NOTE: If your back muscles are extremely tight, resting your head on the floor will be uncomfortable. Use a pillow or some books beneath your head.

3 Repeat this process on your right shoulder using your left hand.

4 Once the balls are positioned correctly, cross your arms over your chest as if you were hugging yourself. Inhale slowly and deeply so that first your abdomen, then your chest, rises with the incoming breath. Relax onto the balls as you exhale. Continue breathing deeply until you feel the balls "sink" into your loosening shoulder muscles.

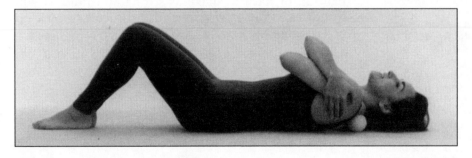

EXPERIENCE NOTES

When activating acupressure points, you will often feel a sensation "radiating" toward adjacent areas of your body. When activating SI-12 you may feel this sensation radiate throughout your neck and shoulders. Don't be alarmed; many people have this reaction to activating SI-12. It occurs with some and not with others and in neither case is it a matter for concern.

SHOULDER VALLEY
SI-10

CHRIS

Chris is a lineman for the Miami Dolphins who happened to be in the training room when I was demonstrating the Acupressure Warmup to one of the trainers. After the demonstration Chris asked if there were points that would work on his shoulders. Shoulder pain and tightness prevented him from lifting one arm beyond parallel to the ground. I showed him the locations of SI-10 (Shoulder Valley), N-UE-14 (Shoulder Mountain) and LU-2 (Pushing Away) and taught him to activate these points. We immediately retested his range of movement. Not only could he raise his arm well above parallel, but he also reported a two-thirds reduction of the pain.

In cases such as Chris's, the more frequently acupressure is applied, the faster the results will arrive. Chris's pain returned after thirty minutes or so but to a lesser degree than before he used the Acupressure Warmup. After the large initial improvement, it is not unusual for the symptom to make its presence known again. This is the optimal time to repeat the acupressure procedure. Chris proceeded in this manner and the time between recurrence of the pain and tension continued to increase until he was entirely free of pain and restriction.

SHOULDER VALLEY is named for the depression that forms when you raise an arm parallel to the ground. SI-10 is located in that depression. The muscles associated with this point are the infraspinatus and the posterior deltoid. These muscles are extremely important for all racquet sports and any throwing motion. Activating this point will relax these muscles and help prevent them from becoming injured.

If there is an affliction of the muscles of this area, you will experience pain or discomfort when you pull your arm backward. Rowing exercises or a one-handed backhand in any racquet sport will be difficult, perhaps painful, or hard to make as strong and fluid as you would like. You may also find it difficult to pick up objects from the ground.

LOCATION
SI-10

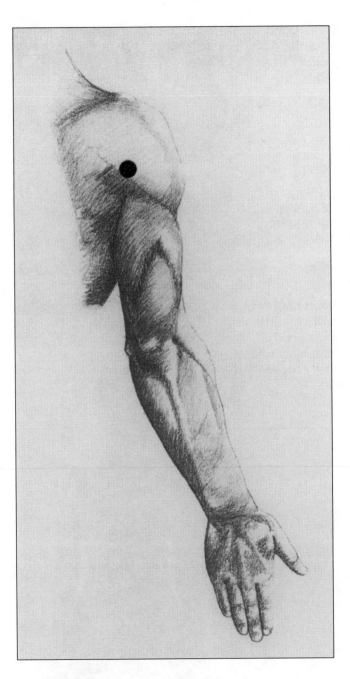

LOCATION

Toward the outside of your body above the crease between your upper arm and body (the Axillary Fold), beneath the large bone found in the depression that forms when your arm is raised.

LOCAL ANATOMY

There are several veins, arteries and nerves in this area: the posterior circumflex humeral artery and vein; deeper, the suprascapular artery and vein; the posterior cutaneous nerve of the arm, the axillary nerve; deeper, the suprascapular nerve. The infraspinatus and posterior deltoid muscles are located here.

HOW TO LOCATE
SHOULDER VALLEY

1 Sit comfortably on your knees and raise your arm until it is parallel to the ground. Place your index finger on the tip of your shoulder.

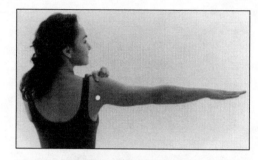

2 Slide your finger over the back of your shoulder until it falls into the depression you will find there.

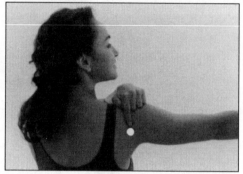

NOTE: When you let your arm fall flat against your side there will be a line between your arm and upper body. This line is known as the axillary fold. This point is located directly above the upper end of this fold.

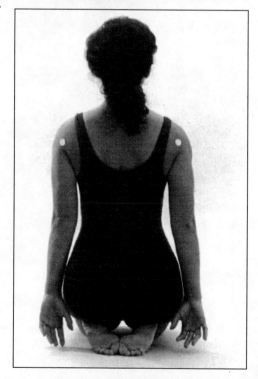

ACTIVATING THE POINT
SI-10

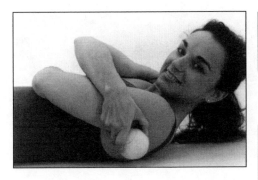

1 When you have finished activating the previous point, SI-12, pick up the tennis ball on your left side with your right hand.

2 Turn your head and shoulders to the left, then place the ball beneath SI-10.

3 Roll onto your left side, easing your weight onto the tennis ball until you feel the achy, activated-point sensation. Breathe deeply and slowly until the ache diminishes.

4 Lie flat, then repeat the exercise on your right side.

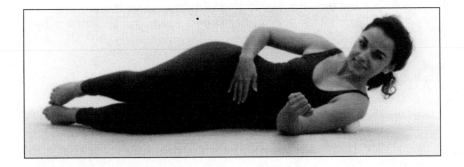

EXPERIENCE NOTES

You will be able to control the amount of pressure applied to the point by how far forward you roll you hips. Don't try to "climb on top of the ball"; you will gain greater control of the activation with less discomfort if you roll your hips.

If the ball squeezes out from under you, it is probably located too far outward.

SHOULDER MOUNTAIN
N-UE-14

BECAUSE OF RECENT clinical successes, N-UE-14 has been added to the list of acupressure points recommended for the shoulder area. It is located on the highest point of the shoulder when the arm is raised and is thus called SHOULDER MOUNTAIN.

When you activate N-UE-14 you affect the deltoid muscle. This is the muscle used to raise your arm to the side. If you have difficulty with this movement, it is likely that your deltoid needs attention and that you will feel some pain in response to pressure at N-UE-14. Activating this point also helps to relax the muscles and tendons associated with this area of your body. As with the last point, SHOULDER MOUNTAIN can be activated to help prevent injuries in racquet sports and all other sports that require throwing motions.

LOCATION
N-UE-14

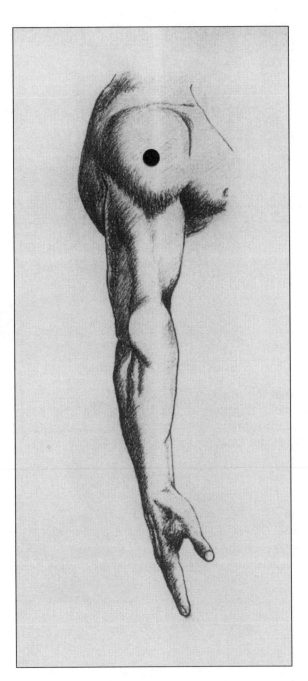

LOCATION

In the middle of the deltoid muscle approximately three inches below the tip of the acromium process of the clavicle.

LOCAL ANATOMY

In the middle of the deltoid muscle. The lateral cutaneous nerve of the arm and, in its deep position, the axillary nerve serve this area. Blood is carried here by the circumflex artery and vein.

HOW TO LOCATE
SHOULDER MOUNTAIN

1   Locate the tip of your shoulder. This is known as the acromium process.

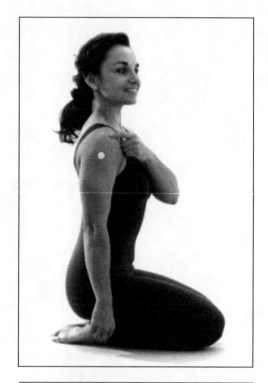

2   Position your hand so that the edge of the index finger lies along the tip of your shoulder. The point is just below the first knuckle of your little finger.

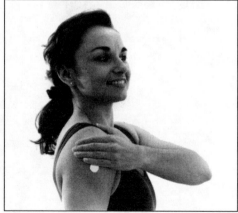

ACTIVATING THE POINT
N-UE-14

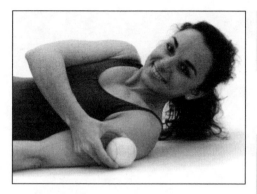

1 After rolling your weight off the tennis ball at the end of the previous exercise, hold one ball in the hand opposite to the side you intend to activate. Place the ball next to the point.

2 Holding the ball in your hand, raise your knees and use their weight to roll your body over the ball.

3 As you relax, breathe deeply and slowly while your body settles onto the balls and the achy sensation subsides.

4 Repeat the entire process on the opposite side.

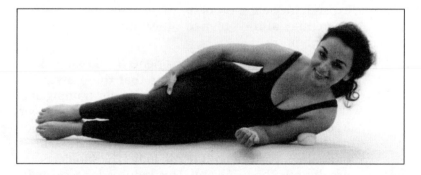

EXPERIENCE NOTES

Govern the amount of pressure applied to the point by how far forward you bend your knees and roll your hips.

If the ball squeezes out from under you, it is probably located too far outward.

To feel the effects of this exercise immediately, raise your arms to the side and notice how much lighter and freer this motion feels.

HOLDING IN FRONT
BL-13

HEATHER

Heather competes in high school lacrosse despite her chronic asthma. Once exertion used to leave her wheezing and short of breath. I taught her to activate "Holding in Front" and "Pushing Away" before she takes the field. Her condition has significantly improved and Heather reports, "I seem to be able to breathe a lot easier and deeper after the acupressure."

THIS POINT IS NAMED HOLDING IN FRONT because the area where you feel tension when you raise your arms in front of your body is where the point is located.

This point is often used clinically for lung problems. The reason for this can be seen by closely watching people who have difficulty breathing. People with respiratory problems often have a posture in which their shoulders are hunched forward. This posture greatly diminishes the ability of their lungs to expand to full capacity. Because their lungs are unable to expand, they are short of breath or easily become dizzy. There may also be myriad other problems related to this condition.

Almost everyone has experienced "choking" in a sporting event. Choking means that the pressure of competition has pushed you beyond your training and skill. Put succinctly, it means that you are blowing your lead and letting the momentum swing in your opponent's favor. Next time you see this, either in yourself or another, observe posture carefully. The shoulders are usually hunched forward. This reduces lung capacity and restricts the amount of oxygen that the muscles receive. If you have a tendency to get too nervous, activate BL-13 frequently before competition. During the competition, between points or plays, be sure to hold your shoulders straight and breathe deeply. While this technique won't cure your case of nerves, it will tone you down and help you focus. Try it! It works!

LOCATION
BL-13

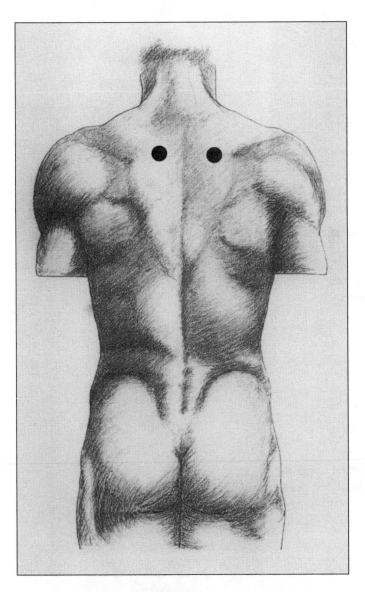

LOCATION

BL-13 is located about two finger-widths toward the outside of the body from the bottom of the third thoracic vertebra.

LOCAL ANATOMY

The medial cutaneous branches of the posterior intercostal artery and vein, as well as parts of the thoracic nerves, are located near BL-13. The trapezius, rhomboid, the posterior inferior serratus and the sacrospinalis muscles form this part of the back.

How to Locate
Holding In Front

1 With your left hand reach over your right shoulder and find the bony ridge.

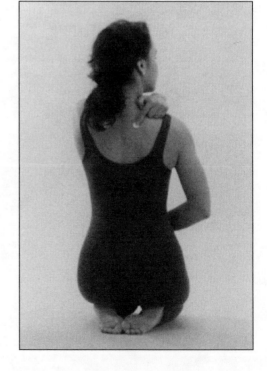

2 Walk your fingers down the ridge toward your spine. After coming off the ridge your fingers will fall into a muscular depression about half way to the spine. This is the point.

3 Repeat this process on the opposite side of the spine to locate left BL-13.

ACTIVATING THE POINT
BL-13

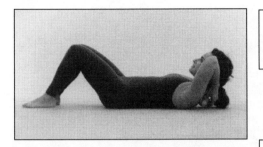

1 After the last exercise, remain on your back for a moment, resting comfortably. Then, raise your shoulders slightly and bend your knees while you reach over your shoulders with both hands to position both balls at BL-13.

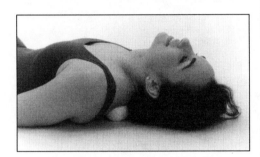

2 Lie back so the balls settle into the muscular depression you found at BL-13.

NOTE: If your back muscles are extremely tight, resting your head on the floor will be uncomfortable. Use a pillow or some books beneath your head.

3 Cross your arms over your body as if hugging yourself and take a slow, deep breath. Exhale slowly as you relax, letting the balls settle further into the muscles of your back.

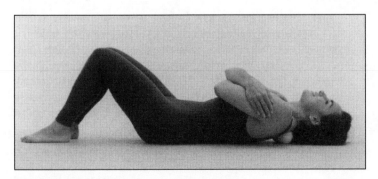

EXPERIENCE NOTES

Once you become familiar with the point locations, you won't need to sit upright to locate them. You will know the locations by experience and you will be able to move from one point to the next very quickly.

If at first you don't feel the point, adjust yourself slightly and the balls will sink into the natural groove between the two large muscles of your back. As always, you will know you have the correct location by the achy sensation.

ROW THE BOAT
BL-15

WHETHER YOU ROW on a machine or on a boat, you will definitely feel the area where this point is located. "Push-pull" exercises like rowing stress this area. This point, like the previous one, is very valuable if you have trouble with "slumping." Slumping not only affects your lungs but also puts an extra strain on your heart. The extra strain on your heart impedes circulation. When your circulation diminishes, every system in your body is affected — muscles, nerves, organs and glands.

Activating this point before a really athletic workout has an excellent result. Experiment with this for yourself. Do what is for you a really hard workout. Keep track of what you could do. In a week, do the same workout again but activate BL-15 first. You will notice that you warm up much faster and that you actually have increased endurance. This point is also excellent for calming yourself before competition.

This point stimulates the rhomboid muscles, which keep your shoulders from hunching forward, the trapezius muscles, which keep your shoulders high, and the sacrospinalis, which keeps your back straight.

LOCATION
BL-15

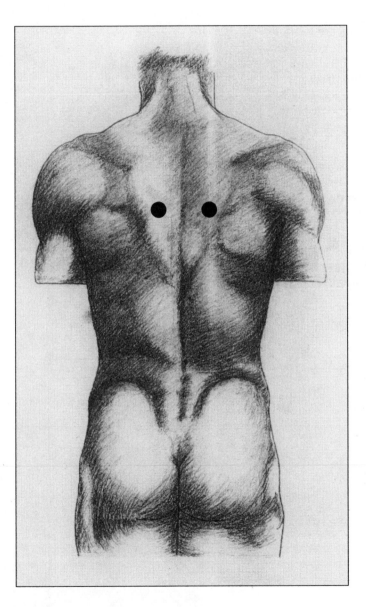

LOCATION

ROW THE BOAT is located in the muscle groove outside the fifth thoracic vertebra.

LOCAL ANATOMY

Branches of the intercostal artery and vein and aspects of the fifth and sixth thoracic nerves and branches are located near BL-15. The trapezius, rhomboid and sacrospinalis muscles form this part of the back.

HOW TO LOCATE
ROW THE BOAT

1 The following few points are located in hard-to-reach places on your back. The position of each point is thus shown in relation to the previous point. The point you are locating is shown by the light colored dot and the previous point is shown by a darker dot.

If you were sitting upright, you would find BL-15 two inches down from the previous point and two inches upward from the lower border of the scapula.

In the second photograph notice how the fingers rest on the upper and lower border of the scapula.

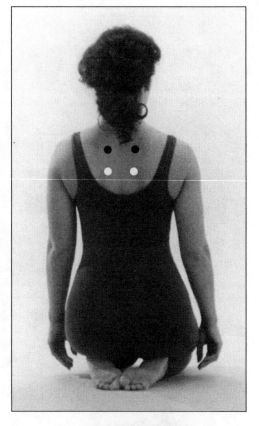

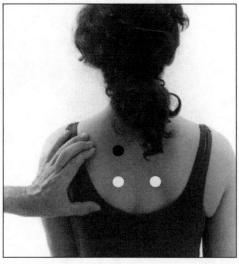

ACTIVATING THE POINT
BL-15

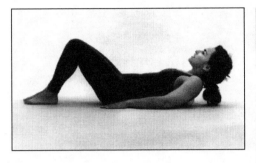

1 Lay your arms to the side and bring your feet closer to your body. Then raise your body slightly taking your weight off the balls, which are still located at the previous point.

2 Push lightly with your feet, rolling the balls down your spine until you feel them to be level with the mid-point of your scapula.

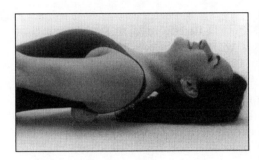

3 Relax onto the balls and rest your hands comfortably on your abdomen.

NOTE: To show you the location in the photograph, the model's arms are lifted. You can leave yours comfortably at your sides.

4 Take a slow, deep breath and exhale slowly as the balls sink into the muscles of your back.

NOTE: If your back muscles are extremely tight, resting your head on the floor will be uncomfortable. Use a pillow or some books beneath your head.

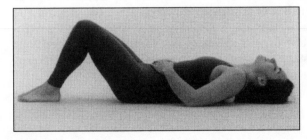

EXPERIENCE NOTES

Because this point is in the center of your upper body there is considerable leverage; be careful not to cause pain. If lowering your weight onto the balls hurts, lessen the pressure by "bridging up" slightly. Remember that nothing should hurt; you should just feel the normal activated-point achiness.

As with all acupressure points, the achiness subsides as relaxation occurs. With this point, the relaxed feeling is particularly strong.

TWISTING AROUND
BL-18

Juan and I frequently traveled together on the professional tennis circuit. At one of the tournaments during a quarterfinal match, Juan's back began to spasm painfully. Although he was able to "guts out" the rest of that match, by evening he was in pain so great that he considered defaulting the semifinals.

Because I felt it could help him, I told Juan not to default but to give my Acupressure routine a chance. I showed him how and he went to work. During the night Juan repeated the warmup at least ten times. In the morning he continued activation of BL-18 (Twisting Around), BL-23 (Lifting Support), BL-25 (Arching the Back), and BL-28 (Stepping Up). By match time he felt well enough to play.

Ten years later Juan is coaching two of the world's top fifty women professional players and continues to use the techniques he learned that day for himself and his players.

BL-18 IS LOCATED in the area of your back that tenses when you twist your upper torso as if to look behind. All movements that involve turning your upper body are enhanced by activating this point.

Along with freeing upper body rotation, BL-18 continues to relax the muscles along the spine. This area of the body is important because it holds great amounts of stress. When people start getting a "hunched back" as they age, it is usually in this area that their troubles begin.

Because all athletes want to exercise throughout their entire life, this particular warmup deserves a place on your list of things to do every day. By keeping the muscles in this area relaxed, your spine will better withstand the unending stress of gravity. The longer your spine stays straight, the longer you will be able to participate in physical activities.

LOCATION
BL-18

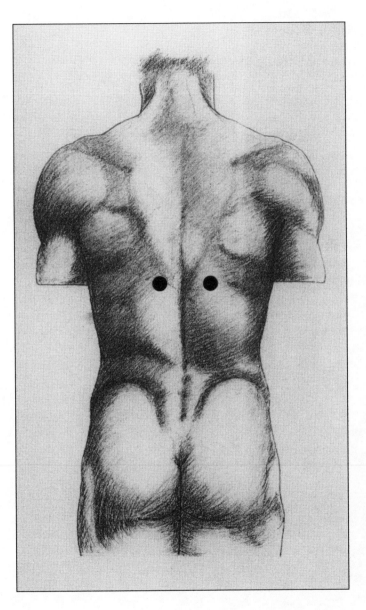

LOCATION

BL-18 is located outward from the lower border of the 9th thoracic vertebra. (Approximately two inches below the bottom of your scapula.)

LOCAL ANATOMY

Branches of the intercostal artery and vein and aspects of the ninth and tenth thoracic nerves and branches are located near BL-18. This area of the back includes the "lats" (latissimus dorsi), the inferior posterior serratus and the sacrospinalis muscles.

HOW TO LOCATE

TWISTING AROUND

1 This point is located relative to the previous point. It is on the same vertical line two inches downward from the bottom of the scapula.

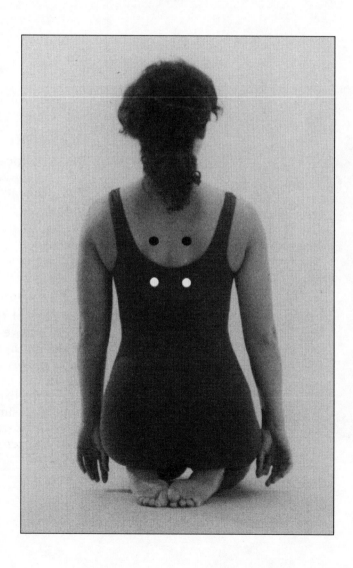

ACTIVATING THE POINT
BL-18

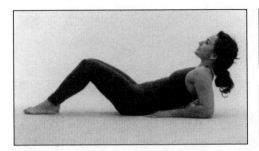

1 Leave the balls at the previous point and bridge up onto your elbows to take your weight off the balls.

2 Push lightly with your feet and roll the balls to BL-18. Straighten your legs and relax, letting the balls sink into the muscles of your back.

NOTE: In the second photograph the arms are raised so that you could see the ball's location. You will be resting lightly on your elbows as you roll the balls to BL-18.

3 Breathe in deeply and exhale slowly, letting the balls sink further into the muscles of your back.

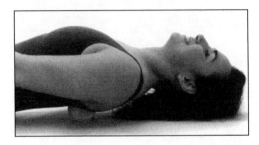

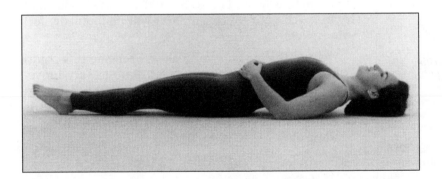

EXPERIENCE NOTES

As with the previous point, you can adjust the pressure by slightly bridging your back. The more you bridge, the less the pressure applied to the point.

When you are in a hurry you can quicken the Acupressure Warmup by starting the balls at BL-13 and rolling them down both sides of your spine in a continuous motion. By rolling the balls over the points you activate each, although less effectively than by resting a while at each point.

LIFTING SUPPORT
BL-23

MARY

Mary's back pain came from stress. She told me, "Every time I get stressed out my back goes out. The last time I couldn't play tennis for six months. My playoffs are in 2 weeks and I really want to play." I promised I would do all I could to get her ready.

Mary didn't like the idea of acupuncture. Although the needles are extremely fine, the "thought" scares some people. Instead, I applied acupressure and heat to BL-18 (Twisting Around), BL-23 (Lifting Support), BL-25 (Arching The Back), BL-28 (Stepping Up) and GB-30 (Jumping Around).

After two weeks of the Acupressure Warmup, she had recovered 80% of her best condition. I advised her not to chance competition but, like most athletes, she played anyway. Her recovery was far enough along that she didn't reinjure her back.

Oh, yes, her team won!

IF THERE WERE ONE most important acupressure point for all purposes, this would be it. Almost everyone you know experiences back pain at times. It is at this point that back pain most often occurs. In acupuncture this point is almost always used for people with back problems.

If you have pain in the lumbar area, bend down slowly to touch your toes. Stop when you feel the tension. Then, activate LIFTING SUPPORT for 30 seconds and try to touch your toes again. You will undoubtedly feel some relief.

As an athlete you should always activate this point! You need a strong lower back for almost every movement that your body is capable of performing. LIFTING SUPPORT is invaluable for loosening your back and is thus important for all sports that require arching or bending over.

LOCATION
BL-23

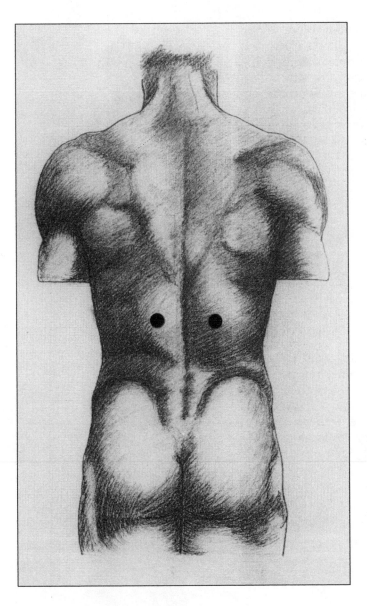

LOCATION

BL-23 is located outward from the lower border of the fourteenth vertebra (lumbar vertebra two) at the level of the navel.

LOCAL ANATOMY

Portions of the second lumbar artery and vein as well as aspects of the first lumbar nerve are found near BL-23. The latissimus dorsi, sacrospinalis and quadratus lumbarum muscles are located here.

HOW TO LOCATE
LIFTING SUPPORT

1 Sit upright and spread your thumb and first finger in a "U" shape. Place the edges of your first fingers along the lower border of your ribs in front and the edges of your thumbs on the lower border of your ribs in back. The tip of your thumb is now just slightly away from the point.

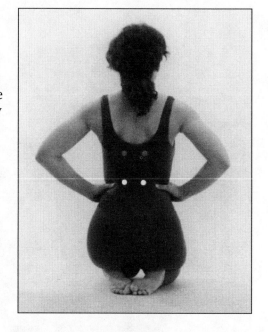

2 Apply slight pressure and move your thumbs toward your spine. You will feel a natural groove between the muscles. The point is now under the tip of your thumb, level with your navel and in line with the previous points.

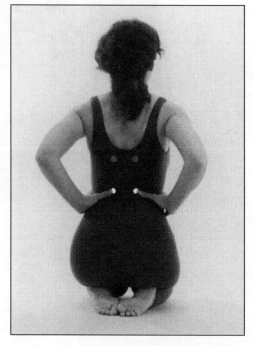

ACTIVATING THE POINT
BL-23

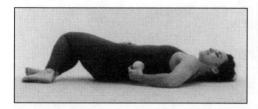

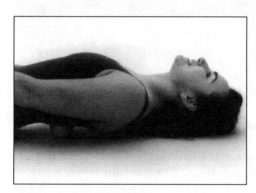

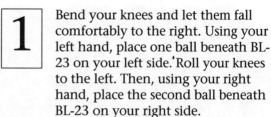

1 Bend your knees and let them fall comfortably to the right. Using your left hand, place one ball beneath BL-23 on your left side. Roll your knees to the left. Then, using your right hand, place the second ball beneath BL-23 on your right side.

2 Straighten and lower your knees slowly, reducing the arch in your back and increasing the weight on the balls until you elicit the now-familiar achy sensation.

3 Breathe in deeply and slowly. Exhale as the balls sink into the muscles of your back.

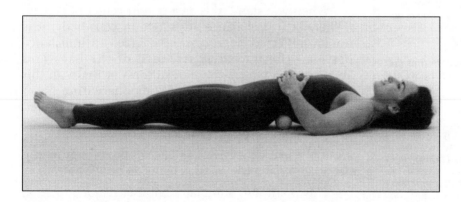

EXPERIENCE NOTES

Once you learn to locate this point by feel, you will want to activate it by rolling the balls down from the previous point. After you find these back points a few times, location becomes easy and the positions feel natural.

ARCHING THE BACK
BL-25

WHEN YOU SIT in a chair and arch your back, the area that tenses is where BL-25 is located. If you stand a lot during the day, this part of your back will often feel stiff and sore. Activating this point will ease the tension. In Oriental medicine this point is closely associated with the large intestine. This is because BL-25 is very beneficial for people who suffer from common problems like diarrhea or constipation.

When you stand, this area is your center of gravity. If there is an imbalance anywhere in your body, it is usually reflected here to some degree. An imbalance between the muscular strength of the back and abdomen is a typical cause of stiffness or injury in this area. Observe the posture of someone with a "beer belly." See how the weight of their abdomen pulls their spine forward in an excessive arch. Their abdominal muscles are too weak and their sacrospinalis muscles are too tense. By activating BL-25 and strengthening the abdominal muscles, back pain can be alleviated.

This point also stimulates another major structural muscle, the psoas major. Tight psoas muscles cause an anterior tilt to the pelvis. This tilt causes the sacrospinalis muscles to shorten and the hamstrings to stretch, which in turn puts the knees in danger of hyper-extension. Because the structural integrity of the entire back depends on the muscles stimulated by this point, ARCHING THE BACK is a very important "preventative point" that should be activated at least once every day.

LOCATION
BL-25

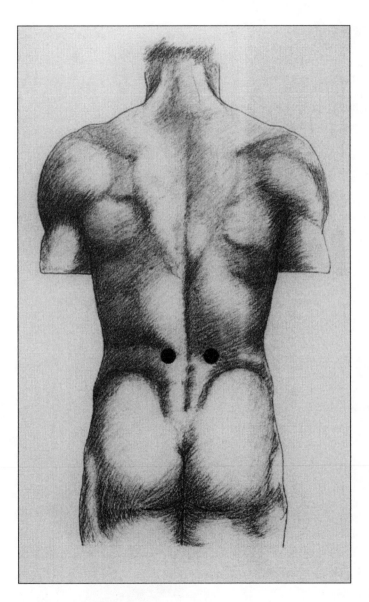

LOCATION

BL-25 is located outward from the lower border of the sixteenth vertebra (lumbar vertebra four), at the level of the iliac crest.

LOCAL ANATOMY

Portions of the fourth lumbar artery and vein and aspects of the third lumbar nerve are located near BL-25. The sacrospinalis, quadratus lumbarum and psoas major muscles comprise this area of the back.

HOW TO LOCATE

ARCHING THE BACK

1 Sit upright on your knees and place your hands on your sides so that the thumb is on your back and your first finger is in front, both following the upper border of your pelvic bone. BL-25 (the white dot) is in line with the previous points (the darker dots) at the level of your waist.

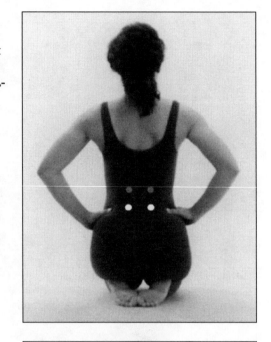

2 Move your thumbs toward the center of your back along the edge of the pelvic bone. BL-25 is in the muscular trough you feel on either side of your spine.

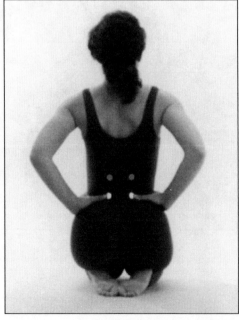

ACTIVATING THE POINT
BL-25

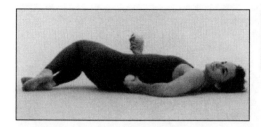

1 Bend your knees and let them fall comfortably to the right. Using your left hand, place one ball beneath BL-25 on the left side. Using your right hand and rolling your knees to the left, place the second ball beneath BL-25 on your right side.

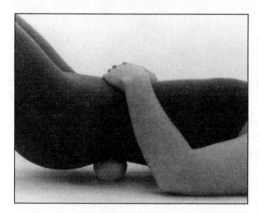

2 Straighten and lower your knees enough to reduce the arch in your back until you elicit the achy sensation.

3 Breath in deeply and slowly. Exhale as the balls sink further into the muscles of your back.

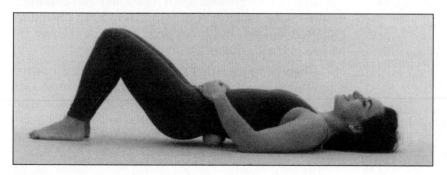

EXPERIENCE NOTES

After activating this, the fifth point on your back, you will notice an increased relaxation in the back area. Compare the difference between the muscle tension in your back and that in your as-yet-unstimulated lower body.

If you feel you have a problem with your lower back and would like to strengthen your abdominal muscles, it is smart to first consult a fitness expert. Because improper abdominal exercise can create problems, it is a very good idea to begin with a well-designed program.

STEPPING UP
BL-28

THIS IS THE AREA of your body that you feel when you hike a steep slope, climb stairs, or work out on a stair climbing machine. An athlete who pursues these activities has the well-developed and rounded buttocks that signify a strong gluteus maximus. STEPPING UP is located on the inner, upper edge of the gluteus maximus. This muscle lifts the thigh upward toward the rear and rotates the hip outward. If it is too tight, it will not only restrict hip and thigh movement but also limit fluidity when walking or running. Activating this point enhances fluidity and helps prevent injuries caused by an overly tense gluteus maximus.

When people finish a stair climbing work out, they often instinctively reach back and apply pressure to this area. The pressure causes the muscles to relax. The Acupressure Warmup applies greater and steadier pressure than is possible with a finger or thumb and has a proportionally greater effect.

When a problem occurs in this area, weakness of the legs and knees is often accompanied by sensations of cold that run up and down the legs and knees. If you experience these feelings, try activating BL-28.

LOCATION
BL-28

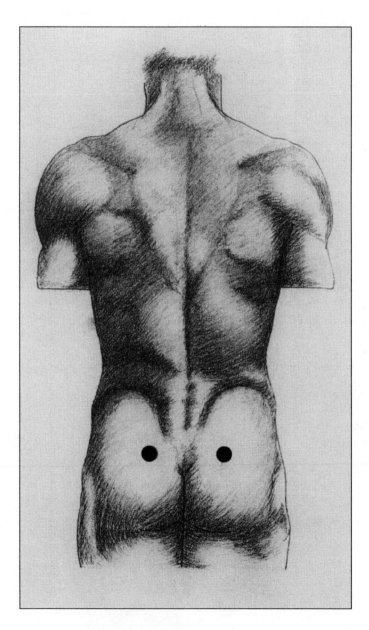

LOCATION

BL-28 is located outward from the lower border of the nineteenth vertebra (sacral foramen two) between the border of the tail bone (sacrum) and the upper pelvis.

LOCAL ANATOMY

Portions of the lateral sacral artery and vein and aspects of the first and second sacral nerves pass near BL-28. The sacrospinalis muscle is located here. STEPPING UP is found at the inner and upper edge of the gluteus maximus.

HOW TO LOCATE

STEPPING UP

1 Sit upright on your knees and place your hands so that your thumbs rest on the dimple formed by the bony protuberance you will find near your sacrum (tail bone).

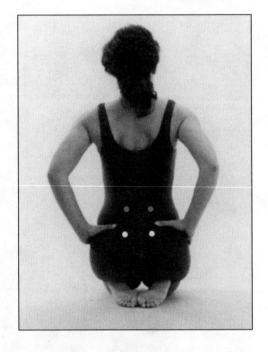

2 Push your thumbs downward until they fall into the depression next to the bony part of your tailbone. BL-28 (the white dot) is in line with the previous points (the darker dots).

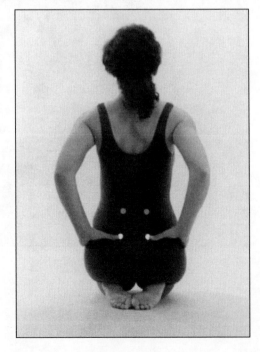

ACTIVATING THE POINT
BL-28

1 Bend your knees only slightly, not as much as you did in the previous exercises. Then, let them fall comfortably to the right. Using your left hand, place one ball beneath BL-28 on the left side. Using your right hand and rolling your knees to the left, place the second ball beneath BL-28 on the right side.

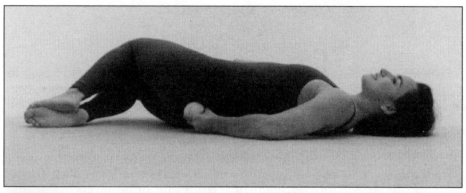

2 Straighten and lower your knees slowly, reducing the arch in your back until you elicit the achy sensation.

3 Breath in deeply and slowly. Exhale as the balls sink deeper into the muscles of your buttock.

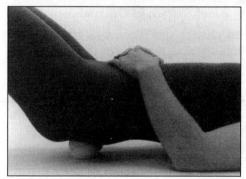

EXPERIENCE NOTES

If your gluteus maximus is particularly strong, you may need to activate both of the BL-28 points one at a time. Apply the extra pressure necessary to elicit the achy sensation by shifting your weight entirely to one side. The increased weight will further activate the point. Again, do not apply so much weight that you cause pain.

JUMPING AROUND
GB-30

CEE CEE

Cee Cee is an aerobics instructor who has been trained in various types of dance. The strain her body has had to endure in these dance positions had led to a chronic hip problem. She told me that sometimes she would be walking along and her hip would "just lock up." When this happened she could not raise her leg to the side or to the front without pain.

After the balls were positioned on the points, Cee Cee's hip would feel better almost immediately. For prevention I recommended that she repeat the process every day. The acupressure points used for this problem are GB-30 (Jumping Around), BL-28 (Stepping Up), ST-31 (Thigh Gate) and GB-31 (Side to Side).

THIS POINT earned its name because it is located in an area that is pivotal for jumping and turning movements. When you bend your knees in preparation for a jump, a round depression will appear on the outside of your buttocks. This is the location of GB-30.

In the Acupressure Warmup, activating this point relaxes the entire hip, buttocks and lower back. Its use for treatment of sciatica and other problems on the outside of the legs is well known in Oriental medicine.

Your ability to change directions quickly is determined by the flexibility and strength of the muscles in this area. Next time you are on the court or playing field, notice where you feel the greatest stress when executing change of direction moves. Typically, you will feel tension from GB-30 all the way down the side of your leg. By activating this point before you play you will not only make these movements more quickly, but also, in the muscular sense, more efficiently.

LOCATION
GB-30

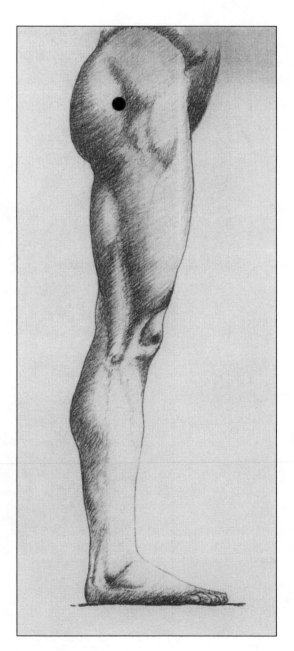

LOCATION

JUMPING AROUND is located in the hip joint. Anatomically, it is located two thirds of the distance along an imaginary line from the sacral hiatus (tip of the tail bone) to the greater trochanter (leg bone).

LOCAL ANATOMY

GB-30 is found near the inferior gluteal artery and vein, the inferior cluneal cutaneous nerve and the inferior gluteal nerve. The sciatic nerve is found here at a deeper level. The gluteus maximus and piriformis muscles are located here.

HOW TO LOCATE

JUMPING AROUND

1 Stand upright and tighten your buttock muscles. You will find GB-30 at the center of the depression that forms on the side of your buttocks.

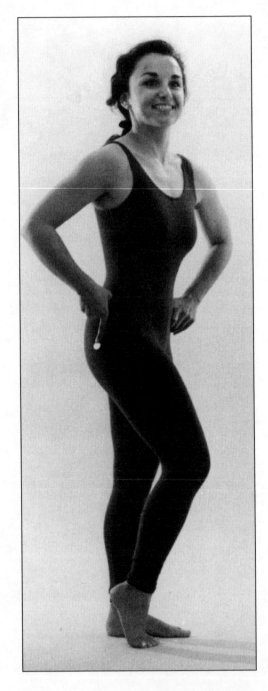

ACTIVATING THE POINT
GB-30

1 Lie flat on the floor with your right knee slightly bent and position a ball at GB-30.

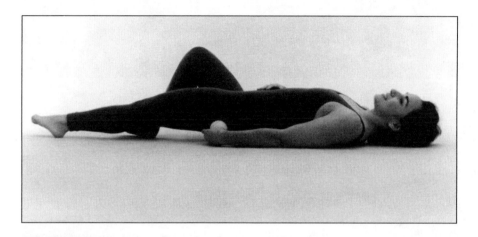

2 Roll your weight onto the ball. Breathe deeply and slowly until the achy sensation subsides.

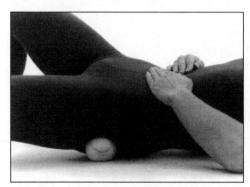

3 Repeat on the opposite side.

EXPERIENCE NOTES

Because the muscles here are many-layered, activating this point will take longer than the points in less densely muscled areas. Leave the balls in place until you feel the surrounding muscles relax.

For additional stimulus turn your body more toward the side to put additional weight over the ball.

For comfort you can place the second ball under your tail bone. This allows you to remain in the correct position longer without bearing your weight constantly on one ball.

UPPER BODY SUPPORT
BL-36

REED

Reed played hockey for the Boston Bruins. During one game he pulled a hamstring muscle. After a week of conventional therapy, he called me for an acupuncture appointment. When I saw him, his range of motion in the pulled hamstring was extremely limited.

Acupoints useful in this type of problem are BL-36 (Upper Body Support) and BL-37 (Sprinter's Valley). After acupuncture his mobility had increased 3 inches in the Sit and Reach Test. When systematically repeated, acupressure techniques will have the same effect as acupuncture for this type of injury. Therefore I demonstrated how to locate and activate these points using the Acupressure Warmup. Reed came for two more treatments and reported that the acupressure "definitely speeded my recovery." He was back in the game the following week.

THIS POINT is located at the junction of the legs and trunk where the weight of your upper body rests. Because your hamstrings originate in this area, this point is extremely useful for treating any hamstring problem.

When someone has back pain, the muscles in their back are often contracted. This contraction causes an upward pull on the pelvic girdle, which puts extra tension on the hamstrings. Activating BL-36 will relax the hamstrings directly and the back muscles indirectly. By relaxing both sets of muscles you allow them to stretch. This reduces the "tug-of-war" between the back muscles and the hamstrings. Your pelvis will then return to a balanced position.

LOCATION
BL-36

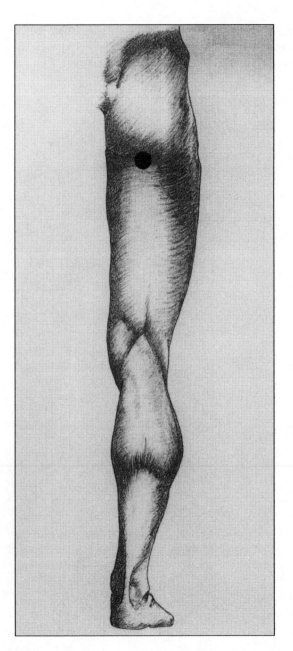

LOCATION

BL-36 is located in the middle of the transverse gluteal fold (the crease between the buttock and thigh).

LOCAL ANATOMY

The artery and vein that run alongside the sciatic nerve, the posterior femoral cutaneous nerve, and deeper, the sciatic nerve, pass through this area. The biceps femoris (hamstring), semitendinosus, gluteus maximus and abductor magnus muscles are all affected by BL-36.

HOW TO LOCATE

UPPER BODY SUPPORT

1 Stand upright reaching behind and beneath your buttock to find the crease. BL-36 is in the center of that crease.

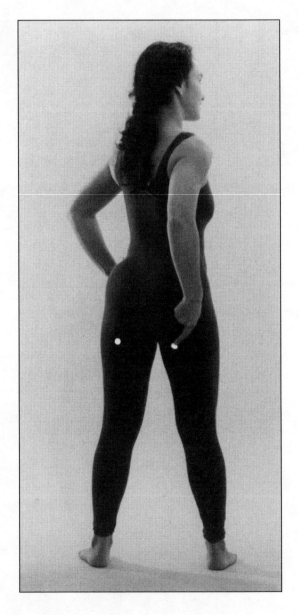

ACTIVATING THE POINT
BL-36

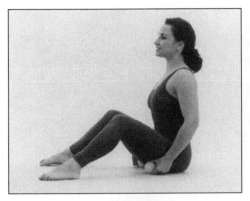

1 Sit with your knees bent and your legs spread at a 45 degree angle.

2 Place the balls beneath both legs at the edge of your buttocks in the center of your hamstring muscles.

NOTE: This point is nearly on the sciatic nerve. If you suffer from sciatica, skip this exercise or try positioning the balls further down your legs.

3 Lean forward and straighten your knees until you feel the achy sensation. Breathe slowly and deeply until the ache subsides.

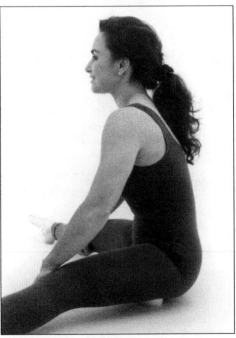

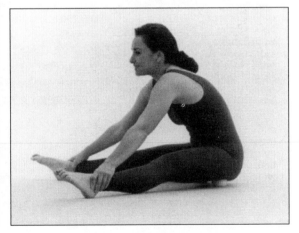

E XPERIENCE NOTES

This point is usually very sensitive to pressure. A strong sensation is fine but don't forget that it should not be painful. You can control the amount of pressure by modifying the angle of knee bend and how far forward you lean.

Some people will feel the sensation from activating this point all the way down to the back of their knees. If this happens to you, and you find the sensation uncomfortable, apply pressure to the back of both knees with your thumbs. This should eliminate the discomfort. If it doesn't, the activation is too strong; bend your knees more and lean forward less.

SPRINTER'S VALLEY
BL-37

SPRINTER'S VALLEY is located in the "valley" between the two large muscles on the back of your legs. These are the biceps femoris and the semitendinosus muscles and are usually very well developed in runners.

Muscle tears and pulls are common in this part of the body. These injuries are caused by the muscular overextension that occurs when you lose your footing or push yourself so hard that you drive these muscles beyond their physical limits. Combined with the previous point, SPRINTER'S VALLEY helps prevent injuries and enhances the loosening of the back muscles begun by activating UPPER BODY SUPPORT.

LOCATION
BL-37

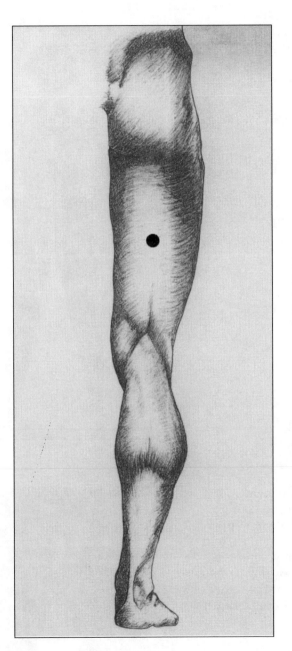

LOCATION

BL-37 is located about six inches below the center of the gluteal fold (the crease between the buttock and thigh).

LOCAL ANATOMY

Branches of the third perforating artery and vein run alongside this point. The posterior femoral cutaneous nerve passes through this area. The muscles here are the biceps femoris (hamstring), semitendinosus and abductor magnus.

HOW TO LOCATE

SPRINTER'S VALLEY

1 Imagine a line between the center of the gluteal fold and the center of the knee crease. BL-37 is on this line, directly below BL-36.

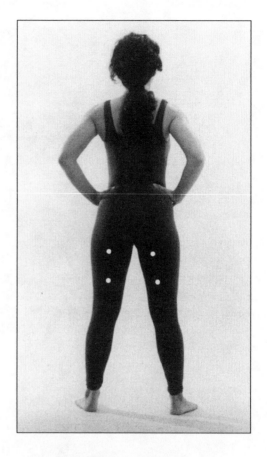

2 While standing, bend down and place both hands behind your leg with the little finger of your upper hand at the edge of the gluteal fold. Put the little finger of your lower hand next to the index finger of your upper hand. BL-37 is in the center of your leg, at the edge of the index finger of the lower hand.

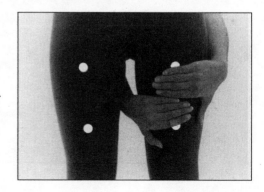

ACTIVATING THE POINT
BL-37

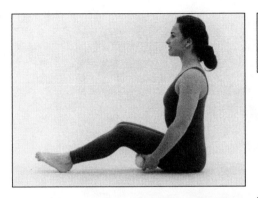

1 Sit with your knees slightly bent and your legs straight in front. Place a ball under BL-37 on both sides.

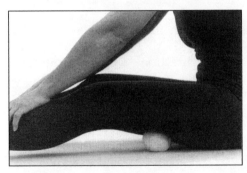

2 Lean forward and straighten your knees until you feel the achy sensation.

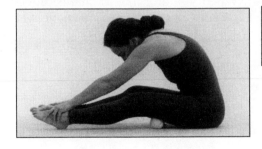

3 Lean further forward as the achy feeling subsides. This provides additional pressure to the point and will increase the relaxation of the hamstring muscles.

EXPERIENCE NOTES

If you have difficulty obtaining the achy feeling, put both balls in the palms of your hands and place them beneath the points. You can apply additional pressure by pushing the balls upward against the points with your hands.

SIDE TO SIDE
GB-31

THIS POINT is located on the part of the body that bears the brunt of all side to side movements and receives the stresses of directional change. Combined with SPRINTER'S VALLEY, SIDE TO SIDE is excellent for muscular problems in the hip area or on the side of the legs.

This point is as important to side-to-side movements as GRAVITY SUPPORT (Exercise 16) is to balance and quick response. Without power and agility in this area you won't be able to change direction as quickly as you otherwise might. When you are slow to change direction, it is easier for your opponents to outmaneuver you.

LOCATION
GB-31

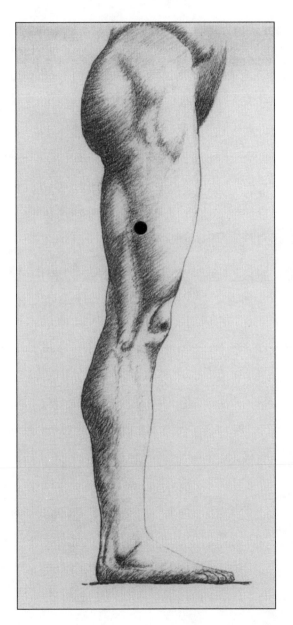

LOCATION

GB-31 is located on the outside of the thigh approximately seven inches above the popliteal crease (knee crease) in a depression between two large muscles.

LOCAL ANATOMY

The muscular branches of the lateral circumflex artery and vein, the lateral femoral cutaneous nerve, and the muscular branch of the femoral artery are located here. GB-31 is found on the vastus lateralis muscle.

HOW TO LOCATE
SIDE TO SIDE

1 Lie flat on your back with your hands and arms flat against your sides; GB-31 is at the tip of your middle finger.

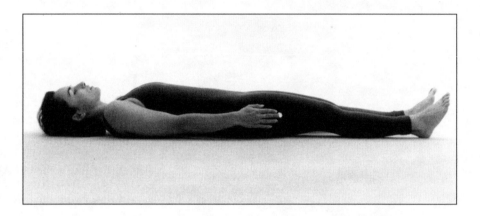

ACTIVATING THE POINT
GB-31

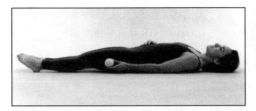

1 Lie flat with one ball in your left hand at the position of GB-31.

2 Bend your knees by moving your feet toward your body while holding the ball at the point.

3 Roll the weight of your legs onto the ball to produce the achy sensation. Breathe deeply and slowly until the ache subsides.

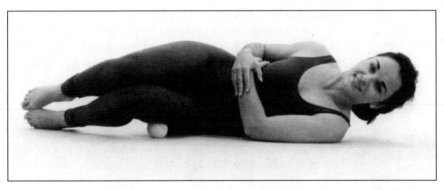

4 Repeat on the opposite side.

EXPERIENCE NOTES

The bend in your knees and the extent that you roll your weight onto the ball will control the pressure applied to the point.

THIGH GATE
ST-31

LOCATED AT THE origin of the sartorius muscle, THIGH GATE has a strong effect on the entire thigh area. In Oriental thought this point is known for its ability to warm the muscles of the thigh region. In this context, "warming" refers to the circulatory increase that activating this point provides.

Because it loosens muscles and increases circulation in the thighs, THIGH GATE is an extremely important point for people who enjoy riding bicycles or exercising on cycling machines. You have probably noticed that cyclists often have strong and well defined thighs. This means that the brunt of the work in cycling is done by this part of the body. Cyclists are well advised to activate this point every day to help prevent injury.

Because bending backward also requires flexibility in the thigh area, this point will be very useful for you if your ability to bridge up is limited. To understand what is meant by "bridge up," see the section on flexibility tests where you will learn to perform a bridge-up test.

LOCATION
ST-31

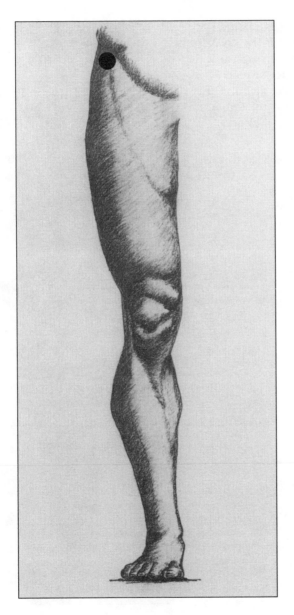

LOCATION

ST-31 is located below the iliac spine in the depression formed when the thigh muscle (sartoris) is flexed.

LOCAL ANATOMY

At a deep level the branches of the lateral circumflex femoral artery and vein traverse this area. The lateral femoral cutaneous nerve is also found here. There are two important muscles in this area, the rectus femoris and sartorius.

HOW TO LOCATE
THIGH GATE

1 Locate the A.S.I.S. (anterior superior iliac spine) by feeling for the bony protrusion that is directly upward from the outside border of your knee cap. If you have trouble locating this protrusion, lie flat on your stomach. The A.S.I.S. is the bone that first touches the floor.

This point, and the two that follow (GRAVITY SUPPORT and BALANCE CENTER), are activated one side at a time because of their location.

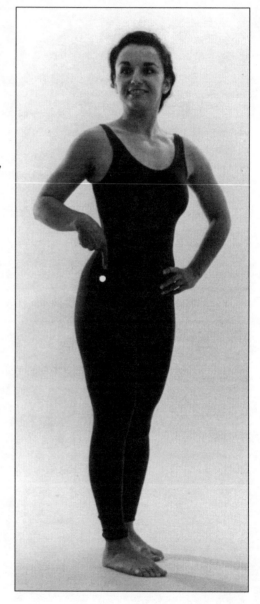

ACTIVATING THE POINT
ST-31

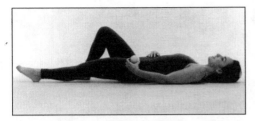

1 Lie down on the floor and position one ball over the depression you feel when you slide your finger slightly outward and downward from the A.S.I.S. (anterior superior iliac spine).

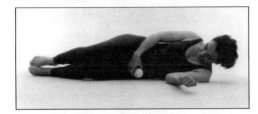

2 Turn onto your side, keeping the ball positioned against ST-31.

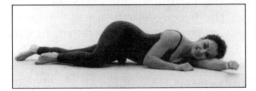

3 Continue turning over until the weight of your body is resting on the ball. Bending the opposite leg at the knee will help keep your body in the proper position.

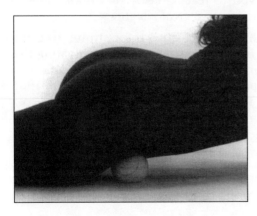

4 Continue to breathe deeply and slowly until the achy feeling subsides.

5 Repeat the process on the opposite leg.

EXPERIENCE NOTES

If the stimulus is too strong or too weak, you can alter the pressure by slightly rotating your hips.

Many people feel the stimulus from activating ST-31 all the way down to the outside part of their knee.

GRAVITY SUPPORT
ST-32

BOB

Bob, a carpenter, always wanted to climb Longs Peak but had put it off for years. On one of his days off we decided to make the hike together. This is an 18 mile round trip and, while it is well enough traveled for an amateur climber to undertake safely, it is a very demanding climb in terms of physical labor.

Since Bob hadn't been hiking or exercising, his legs began cramping on the way up. I taught him about the acupoints which are known to relieve cramps. These are KI-1 (Balance Center) and BL-57 (Mountain Support). These points alone are usually enough to relieve leg cramps. In Bob's case I also applied acupressure to ST-31 (Thigh Gate), ST-32 (Gravity Support), and LV-9 (Scissors Kick).

Within a couple of minutes Bob was hiking again, pain free. Occasionally, the cramps would return and he would repeat the process on his own with the same results. He made it to the top!

BALANCE IS the common denominator of all sports. Balance gives you agility, momentum, strength, finesse, power, quickness and coordination. The lower your center of gravity, the better your balance. To lower your center of gravity you must crouch down. In this position, your thigh muscles do most of the work. This is why the thigh muscles are so important in sports. Crouching not only lowers your center of gravity but also prepares you to react quickly. If you are able to react quickly, you have a great advantage.

ST-32 is the point of choice for stimulating the thigh muscle. In fact, the stimulus from activating this point is so strong that you will need to be careful not to let it become painful. Because of the muscular relation of the thighs to the knees, GRAVITY SUPPORT is also a good choice for people with knee problems.

Location
ST-32

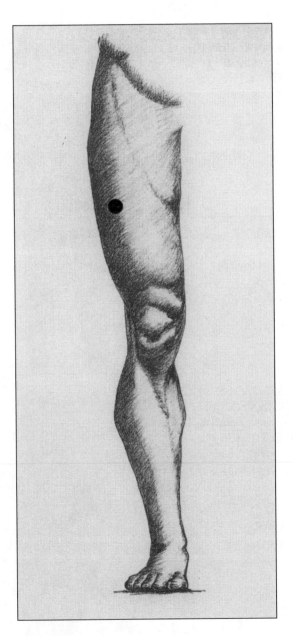

Location

ST-32 is located in a fleshy prominence six inches upward on an imaginary line from the outer and upper border of the patella (kneecap) toward the A.S.I.S. (Anterior Superior Iliac Spine).

Local Anatomy

ST-32 is found near branches of the lateral circumflex femoral artery and vein, and the anterior and lateral femoral cutaneous nerves. The rectus femoris and vastus lateralis muscles are located here.

HOW TO LOCATE

GRAVITY SUPPORT

1 Position your index finger of your left hand on the outer and upper edge of your right kneecap. Put your other index finger on your A.S.I.S. (which you found for the previous point, THIGH GATE).

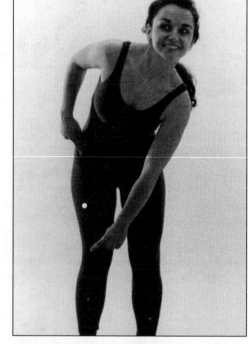

2 Notice the muscular trough on the line between your two index fingers. The point is located on this imaginary line approximately 6 inches upward from the knee cap.

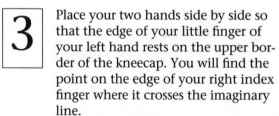

3 Place your two hands side by side so that the edge of your little finger of your left hand rests on the upper border of the kneecap. You will find the point on the edge of your right index finger where it crosses the imaginary line.

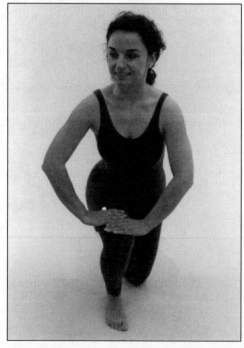

ACTIVATING THE POINT
ST-32

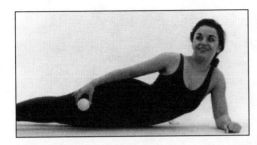

1	Position the ball over ST-32.

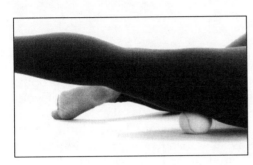

2	Roll over onto the ball and bend the knee of the opposite leg.

3	Breathe deeply and slowly as the ache subsides.

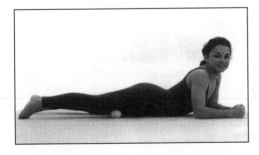

4	Repeat on opposite leg.

EXPERIENCE NOTES

When activating this point, put some of your weight on the opposite leg (the one with the bent knee). This will reduce the strong stimulus that frequently occurs when ST-32 is activated.

Try touching your heel to your buttocks before and after activating this point; you should notice a big improvement.

BALANCE CENTER
KI-1

IN ORIENTAL martial arts and medicine, KI-1 is known as the primary balance point of the whole body. When you stand upright, the entire weight of your body is centered here. Structurally, BALANCE CENTER is very important for keeping your body aligned with gravity. If there is an imbalance in this alignment, it will show as pressure pain at KI-1 and as muscle pains, strains and cramps throughout your body. If you are structurally imbalanced, your muscular system will be imbalanced as well.

This point is very useful for athletes because it can stop muscular cramping anywhere in the body. By activating this point you will not only help yourself adjust to gravity physically but also help alleviate muscular imbalances that could lead to cramping. Another benefit is that KI-1 can eliminate the dizziness that occurs with heat stroke.

LOCATION
KI-1

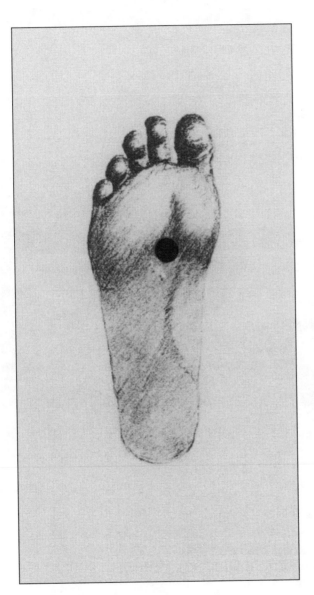

LOCATION

KI-1 is located one third of the distance from the base of the toes to the back of the heel in a depression on the sole of the foot.

LOCAL ANATOMY

The plantar arch is beneath this point, and the second common plantar digital nerve passes through this area.

HOW TO LOCATE

BALANCE CENTER

1 Cross one leg over the other knee so that you can see the bottom of your foot.

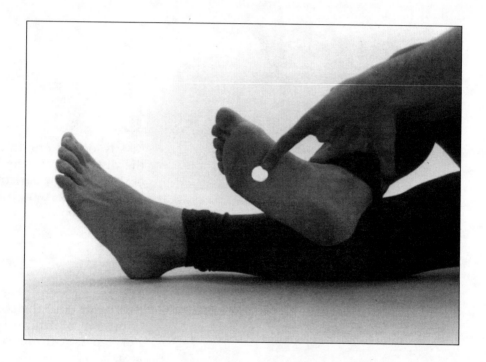

2 Locate the depression in the center of the sole about one third of the length of your foot from the base of your toes.

ACTIVATING THE POINT
KI-1

1 Place a ball on the floor, putting the depression in the sole of your foot on the ball.

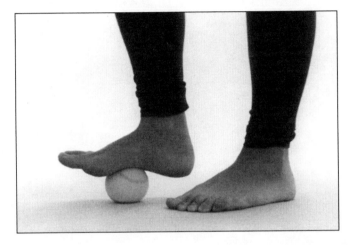

2 Slowly shift your weight onto the ball until you feel the achy sensation. Breathe slowly and deeply until the sensation subsides.

3 Repeat on the opposite foot.

EXPERIENCE NOTES

The combination of this point with BL-57, MOUNTAIN SUPPORT, is excellent for relieving leg cramps associated with sports that require a lot of leg work.

If you don't receive enough stimulus on this point using a tennis ball, try using something harder like a baseball or golf ball. This is the only point where it is all right for everyone to use a harder ball. On the other points the additional pressure might be too painful.

PRESSURE EXERCISES

PUSHING AWAY
LU-2

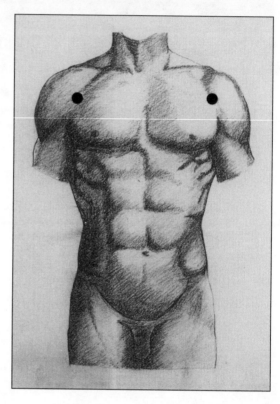

PUSHING AWAY takes its name from its location on the pectoral muscles. These muscles are used to push away from the body, for example, when doing push-ups. Activating this point not only relaxes and strengthens the pectoral muscles but is also very beneficial for asthmatics. Its effects will be appreciated by any athlete with a respiratory problem. If you ever have difficulty taking a deep breath after heavy exertion, activate this point. LU-2 has a moderating effect that allows the lungs to expand and take in more air. Remember that BL-13 has a similar effect on the lungs. Thus activating LU-2 and BL-13 can be very beneficial for those suffering from respiratory limitations.

Another muscle this point affects is the anterior deltoid. The anterior deltoid lifts your arm upward in front of your body. It also helps rotate your shoulders forward. If you have problems with either of these movements, PUSHING AWAY is an important point for you.

LOCATION

On the chest, immediately below the outside extremity of the clavicle about six inches outward from the midline.

LOCAL ANATOMY

The cephalic vein, the thoracoacromial artery and vein; inferiorly, the axillary artery; the intermediate and lateral supraclavicular nerve, the branches of the anterior thoracic nerve and the lateral cord of the brachial plexus are located in this area. The point is located near the pectoralis major and anterior deltoid muscles.

LOCATION AND ACTIVATION
PUSHING AWAY

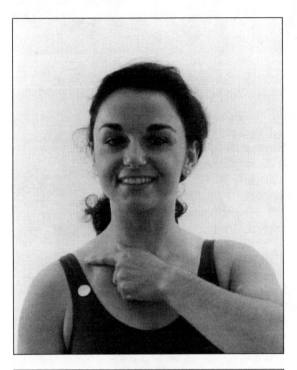

1 Using your left hand to locate right LU-2 (or vice-versa), slide your index finger along your clavicle until it comes to rest in a cleft at the end of the bone.

2 The point is located in the depression at the edge of the chest muscle straight down from this cleft.

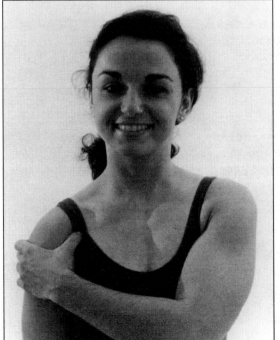

3 Press with your thumb to produce the achy sensation. To apply greater pressure you can grasp the outside of your arm and squeeze, utilizing the strength of your hand.

4 Repeat on the opposite side.

HOLDING FIRM
LI-11

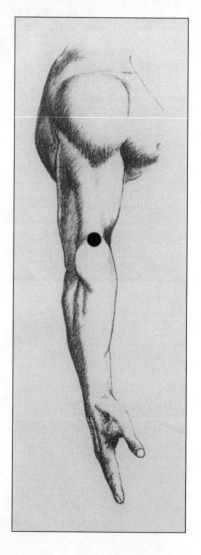

HOLDING FIRM affects all of the muscles and tendons used to grip, hold and flex your hand and arm. This point is located at the origin of the extensor carpi radialis and, on the lateral side, the brachioradialis muscles. These muscles are primarily responsible for gripping and flexing. They are often overworked in sports like tennis, golf and baseball where grip strength is important. Because of the strain placed on these muscles, this area of the arm is vulnerable to tendonitis (tennis elbow). If you have experienced the tense, strained feeling that signals the early stages of this problem, regularly activating LI-11 will help relieve it and may prevent its further development.

LOCATION

When the elbow is flexed, the point is in the depression at the lateral end of the transverse cubital crease (elbow crease) at the highest point of the muscle.

LOCAL ANATOMY

The branches of the radial recurrent artery and vein, the posterior antebrachial cutaneous nerve and, deeper on the medial side, the radial nerve are located here.

LOCATION AND ACTIVATION

HOLDING FIRM

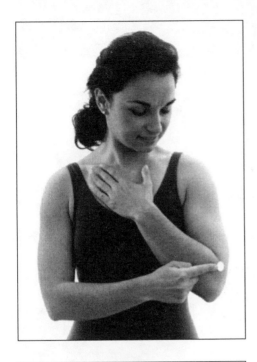

1 Place your hand on your chest as shown.

2 Find the crease at your elbow. LI-11 is located at the end of this crease on the highest point of the muscle.

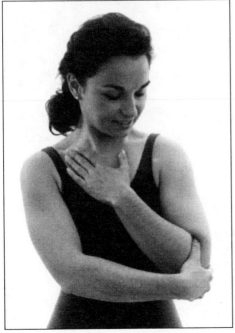

3 Apply pressure to the point with your thumb until you produce the achy sensation.

SCISSORS KICK
LV-9

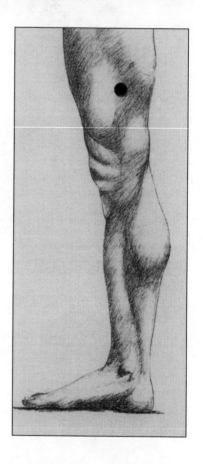

IN GYMNASTICS when splits are performed, or in karate when the side kick is executed, it is thigh strength and flexibility that is required. Certain dance movements and the ability to ride a horse also depend on the large muscles of the inner thigh. In sports that require lateral movement, for example, tennis, soccer and basketball, players depend on these muscles for the stability of their knees.

It is balance that the athlete requires. Strength and flexibility are equally important. For example, if one of your sartorius muscles is weak and the other strong, the pelvis will rotate slightly, straining other areas of your body, particularly your back. You can determine if these muscles are imbalanced when you apply pressure. The side that is less healthy will be more sensitive to pressure. If you find you have this problem, activate SCISSORS KICK as often as possible to help restore your balance.

LOCATION

LV-9 is located between the two large muscles on the inner face of the thigh, about four inches above the knee.

LOCAL ANATOMY

On the lateral side and deep are the femoral artery and vein. Also located here are the anterior femoral nerve and the superficial branch of the medial circumflex femoral artery. The point is located on the pathway of the anterior branch of the obturator nerve. The point is between the sartorius and the vastus medialis muscles.

LOCATION AND ACTIVATION

SCISSORS KICK

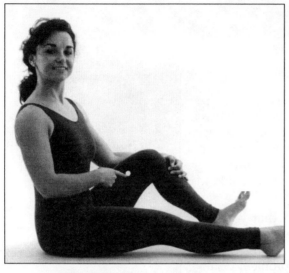

1 Sitting, bend one knee at a 90 degree angle and flex your foot upward.

2 Slide your thumb into the depression that is present between the two large muscles of your inner thigh, four inches up from the inside of the knee.

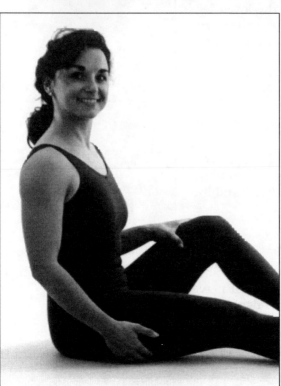

3 Hold your leg from above with your thumb resting in the depression and apply pressure to the point.

MUSCULAR POWER
GB-34

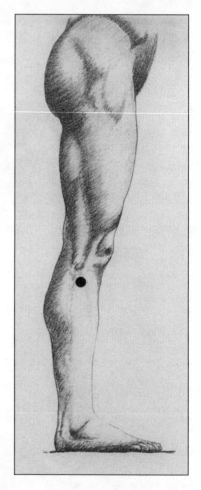

IN ACUPUNCTURE theory this point is thought to affect every muscle in the body. It is known for increasing the strength and endurance of the entire muscular system in general and the leg muscles in particular. Activating this point helps warm up the area of the leg which is responsible for jumping, running, and side to side movement.

Shin splints are a common problem that you can help prevent by activating this point before participating in activities that cause stress or "pounding" in the shin area. Ankle sprains are an athletic problem occurring because of muscular imbalances in the lower leg. When an ankle is sprained, MUSCULAR POWER will be sensitive to pressure. When GB-34 is then activated, some of the pain and stiffness that accompanies the sprain will be alleviated, and recovery time shortened.

LOCATION

GB-34 is found one inch below the knee in a depression on the outer face of the shin, between the two bony protuberances which are the heads of the fibula and the tibia.

LOCAL ANATOMY

The inferior lateral genicular artery and vein are found here. This point is where the common peroneal nerve splits into the superficial and deep peroneal nerves. The muscles located here are the peroneus longus and the extensor digitorum longus.

LOCATION AND ACTIVATION

MUSCULAR POWER

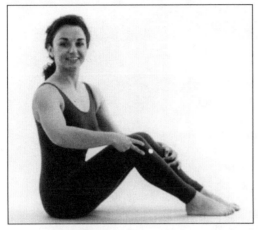

1 Sitting with your knees bent, locate the two bony protrusions on the lower outside of the knee area. Place your index finger and middle finger on these protrusions.

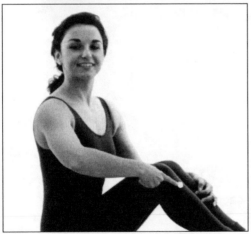

2 Slide your index finger into the notch between these two protrusions, then slide slightly down until your finger falls into a depression. This depression is the location of GB-34.

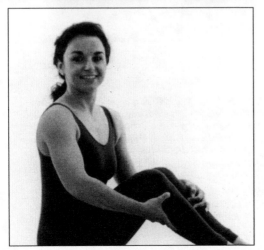

3 Activate the point with your thumb, applying pressure to elicit the achy sensation.

MOUNTAIN SUPPORT
BL-57

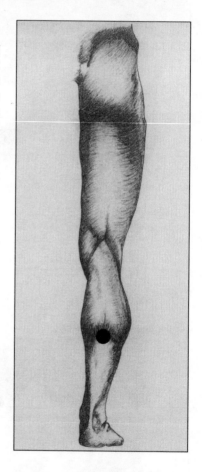

WHEN mountain climbing, running or participating in any sport where your foot must flex and extend, your gastrocnemius muscle (the calf muscle) does most of the work. If you have trouble raising your heel off the ground and pointing your toe, you probably have a problem with the gastrocnemius. Activating BL-57 should help. Tightness of the Achilles tendon can also be alleviated and prevented by activation of this point. Another important quality of MOUNTAIN SUPPORT is that it will help stop muscle cramps anywhere in the leg.

LOCATION

Directly below the calf where the muscle divides.

LOCAL ANATOMY

The small saphenous vein and the medial sural cutaneous nerve; deeper, the posterior tibial artery and vein, and the tibial nerve are located here. The gastrocnemius and soleus are the major muscles in this area.

BILL

Bill is in his 40's. In high school he was unbeatable in the mile. Twenty years later he renewed his interest in competitive running. Because of the amount of time he has been away from running, it was no surprise that Bill developed many minor injuries as soon as he began a training routine. Most of these injuries would heal by themselves. However, one particular injury kept getting worse and worse. Two months after he had injured his Achilles tendon in a race it still hadn't healed.

The best acupressure point for this problem is BL-57 (Mountain Support). It is easy to use finger pressure for this point, so all I needed to do was show him how much pressure he should use — enough to cause an achy feeling but not enough to cause pain.

The following week, during a company 10 kilometer race, he beat his current best time by almost 52 seconds. He told me after the race that his Achilles tendon had felt fine throughout the race.

LOCATION AND ACTIVATION
MOUNTAIN SUPPORT

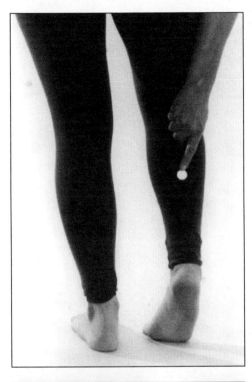

1 When you stand with your heel raised off the floor, BL-57 is located at the tip of the inverted v-shaped calf muscle.

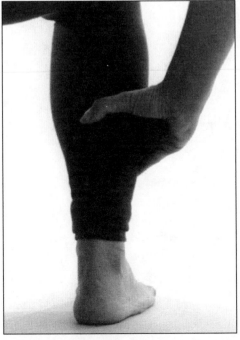

2 Grasp your leg from the side with your thumb on this point and your fingers on the front of your leg. Squeeze until you elicit the achy sensation. Occasionally this point is very sore. If this is the case for you, begin with light pressure, increasing gradually until the soreness is alleviated.

MERIDIAN STRETCHING
EXERCISES

INTRODUCTION TO STRETCHING

T HE STRETCHES PRESENTED HERE are adaptations of exercises that developed in many Oriental arts. Some of the positions are similar to yoga postures and some are similar to the stretching exercises athletes use. The important thing to remember about these stretches is that they are to be done with a different focus — an inner awareness of how the muscles feel instead of a drive toward physical strain.

Although these exercises are presented here only for athletic preparation, several Oriental experts have developed meridian stretches for complex problems. Yoshio Manaka, M.D., perhaps Japan's most prolific and inventive Oriental medical expert, developed diagnostic and treatment systems based on meridian stretching. By changing the body posture and looking for changes of acupoint reactivity, Dr. Manaka was able to predict the usefulness of treatments even while they were in progress. Shizuto Mazunaga, a Japanese massage specialist, developed an entire mind-body exercise system from stretching exercises. In Mazunaga's system, coordinated imagery, breathing and meridian stretching are used for self-treatment and self-development. Dr. Hashimoto, a famous Japanese physician, used stretching to balance the body. For example, Dr. Hashimoto would note which leg was longer and give the patient a stretch-like exercise that would bring both legs into balance. With this method he was able to resolve many people's long-standing problems.

All these systems share a common understanding. The human body reacts to the inevitable daily stresses and strains by becoming imbalanced. This imbalance eventually leads to physiological and anatomical malfunction. Thus the idea behind these exercises is not that you will physically manipulate your body by force but that you will develop an awareness of equilibrium. By stretching away tension and opening your body's natural lines of communication, you will develop the finer sensitivity and greater control that athletics, fitness and injury prevention require.

For each stretch there are instructions on how to get into the proper position. There are also regular reminders of the importance of breathing correctly throughout the entire exercise. Breathing is extremely important in any exercise routine and these stretches are no exception. The entire time you are moving into the posture shown in the photos you should be inhaling slowly and deeply. Once you get to the point of tension in each exercise, you should hold the stretch for a moment, then exhale completely. This is all that is needed to activate the meridians. However, if time permits, you can continue the stretch and gain a greater advantage.

If you have time to continue the stretch, begin as usual. Then, after reaching the first point of tension, slowly and carefully reach for a second, new point of tension. Reach, don't force! Once you reach this new point, take a slow, deep inhalation. Hold the inhalation for a moment then exhale completely. This can be continued for up to five minutes. Be attentive! When you inhale, you will feel increased tension along the meridian. When you exhale, you will feel this tension decrease.

By doing this longer version of the meridian stretches, you will develop an intuitive sense of your muscles and will be more likely to experience the "streaming" sensation associated with opening your meridians. However, even if you have no time for the second stage stretch, the basic routine will be effective in less than five minutes.

To understand these stretches think of a meridian as a communication link. Meridians connect every aspect of physiological and anatomical function to every other aspect. Thus the meridian system is like a telephone network. There are major phone lines connecting major cities. From these major phone lines secondary lines branch to smaller cities. By connecting various lines, any two parties anywhere can talk to one another. Without this ability to communicate our entire society would suffer.

The same is true of your body. It is vastly more flexible than any computer, transmitting and receiving exponentially more messages than are carried by all the phone companies in the world. To function as a human, every part of the body needs information about every other part. The meridians are the main lines of communication. If these lines of communication are healthy, the entire system works harmoniously. If these lines of communication are damaged or inefficient, some messages may arrive late, garbled, or not at all and the entire system will suffer directly or indirectly.

To keep these communications links open we must use them. By stretching and contracting the meridians every day, you will develop the suppleness necessary to keep your system in balance. Therefore, if the course of the meridian isn't stretched or otherwise activated, some form of impairment will appear along the path of the meridian.

While describing the meridians, I often use the word "sinew." I use this word to emphasize that part of the meridian concept that refers less to a physical aspect of your body and more to your ability to stretch and contract, push and pull. In effect, sinew is the combined ability of all the anatomical parts, mental and physiological functions that govern your expansive and contractive ability in particular body areas. It is easier to feel this for yourself than it is to explain. When moving into the stretch postures you will feel certain lines of tension. These lines of tension are typically the pathways of the meridian system. The muscles, flesh and ligaments that more or less follow these paths are the sinew.

When you do these stretches correctly, you should begin to feel a "streaming" sensation. This sensation will move up and down the line of tension and is the result of activating the sinew portion of the meridian. This is the feeling you want! If you experience any pain or discomfort, it means that you are over-stretching.

Meridian impairments can sometimes be inferred from the physiological and anatomical symptoms which I have listed in the introduction to each stretch. While looking over the list of symptoms associated with each meridian you may find that the lists for one or two meridians include most of your symptoms. If this is the case, it could be an indication that this meridian is imbalanced. Spending more time on the stretches associated with those meridians could prove beneficial for your overall health.

Each meridian is related to and, in English, is named for one of the body's organs. These meridian names help label the acupoints and, at times, remind us of therapeutic relationships. However, keep in mind that these meridian names shouldn't be confused with, or compared to, the ideas of body organs you learned in school. In other words, discovering a meridian imbalance isn't evidence of a major problem with a vital organ. Think of a meridian imbalance as a less-than-ideal condition, an athletic limit you will overcome, not a diagnosis of disease.

The meridians discussed in this book are all "bilateral." That is, there is one pathway on each side of your body. Some of the postures stretch both sides at once, others require a change of position, a two-step stretch. Stretches requiring a position change are noted in the "How to Stretch" section.

How to Use This Section

These stretches help solidify the benefits of the Acupressure Warmup. They also help integrate whatever fitness exercise you now use into a broader and more useful program. For example, you might begin with the warmup exercises for ten minutes, move on to stretches for ten minutes, then finish an hour workout with aerobic training.

Each of the 12 stretches is presented in two units:

Instructions for performing the stretch.

Instructions for monitoring your progress.

Like the warmup exercises, the stretches should not hurt. You can abbreviate, select the most important stretch for you, and customize the program for yourself.

How to Stretch

These stretches are not meant to be forced. Unlike conventional stretches, these exercises are part of listening to your body, not a challenge to bend more and faster. If you are interested in longer and more complex programs, there are other Oriental exercise systems known as "Tai Chi" or "Qi Gong" that combine bending, stretching, specific postures and motions into dance-like martial arts. There are references in the reading list.

The Acupressure Warmup stretches have been selected to activate the acupuncture meridians, not to manipulate your anatomy. Begin the stretches after the exercises. When you do the stretches, listen to your body just as you did by concentrating on the changes occurring in the point and surrounding muscles. Pull the muscles you are stretching like an elastic band, but don't create pain or a lot of tension.

A good time to work on mental preparedness is during the stretches. For example, many professional athletes work with sports psychologists who help them with visualized images. Even a beginning athlete can do something similar. Think, for example, of your performance as you would like it to be, or imagine your golf stroke when you have it perfected. Even imagining yourself as calm, cool and collected in the midst of a tight match can be an uplifting experience. Concentrating on the physical feeling of the stretch and how much more flexible you are becoming will also help.

Progress with Stretches

With these stretches you don't so much measure progress as feel it. The first time you do the stretches, take your time, be sensitive to your limits, and pay attention to how you feel. You are activating meridians, something you can think of as improving your body's internal communications system. As your built-in sensitivities develop, you will respond to the stretching with greater relaxation and a sense of well-being.

LUNG MERIDIAN

THE MAIN MERIDIAN and sinew channel associated with the lungs proceeds from the chest to the shoulder and down the outside of the arm to the thumb.

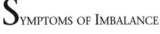

SYMPTOMS OF IMBALANCE

- Pain or weakness when doing push ups
- Respiratory problems
- Hunched shoulders
- Pain or stiffness between the shoulder blades
- Lack of stamina

HOW TO STRETCH

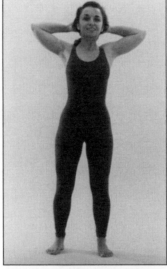

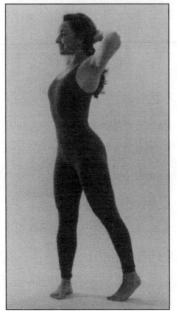

1 Stand comfortably with your legs about shoulder width apart and clasp both hands behind your head.

2 Breathe in deeply and slowly while you turn at the waist as if to look as far to the right as you can.

NOTE: allow your right heel to come off the ground when turning.

3 When you feel tension, hold your position and exhale completely.

4 Repeat this process on the opposite side.

LARGE INTESTINE MERIDIAN

THE LARGE INTESTINE meridian and sinew begin at the index finger and run upward on the outside of your arm, elbow and upper arm. The pathway crosses over your shoulder and neck to end near your mouth at the side of your nose.

SYMPTOMS OF IMBALANCE

- Tennis elbow
- Inability to raise your arm
- Pain or stiffness when turning your head
- Lack of physical strength

HOW TO STRETCH

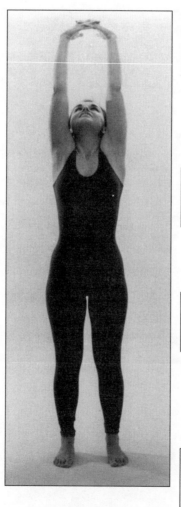

1 Stand straight with your feet about shoulder length apart.

2 Interlock the fingers of your hands.

3 Stretch your hands above your head while looking upward.

4 As you feel the tension, hold your position for a moment, then exhale completely.

STOMACH MERIDIAN

THE STOMACH MERIDI-AN and sinew is long and complex. It begins at the side of the nose, ascending past the inner edge of your eye. It then descends past your lips to your chin. From here it passes upward again through the jaw to the front of your ear. Here, the meridian branches to several places on your face. The main line of the meridian descends through your trunk in line with your nipples, turning inward toward the navel as it continues downward to your thighs. It then passes over your knees and down the outside front of your lower leg to cross the top of your foot and end at your second toe.

SYMPTOMS OF IMBALANCE

- Tension or pain in the middle of your back
- Tension in your shoulders
- Difficulty doing situps
- Wrist or ankle inflexibility
- Shin splints
- Jaw pain
- Frontal headaches

HOW TO STRETCH

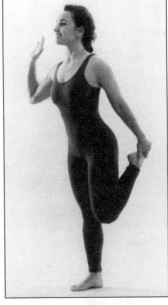

1 Stand straight with your feet about shoulder length apart.

2 Raise your right hand above and in front of your body with your palm facing forward.

3 Raise your left leg by holding your left foot in your left hand.

4 Breathe in deeply and slowly while you stretch both your right arm and your left leg upward and outward.

5 When you feel the tension, hold your position for a moment, then breathe out completely.

6 Relax; repeat on the opposite side.

SPLEEN MERIDIAN

THE CHANNEL named for the spleen begins at your big toe and follows the border between lighter and darker skin which you will find on the inward edge of your foot. Then, passing in front of the ankle to the inside back of your leg, the pathway rises up your inner thigh and zig-zags along your groin and lower abdomen. From there it rises up the front of your chest toward the outside. At about the level of your armpits it turns inward toward your neck where it follows your esophagus inside and upward to end at the base of your tongue.

SYMPTOMS OF IMBALANCE

- Pain or stiffness on the inner side of your knee or lower leg
- Pain or stiffness on the inner part of your ankle
- Pain or stiffness in the mid-back region
- Injuries in your groin area
- Poor digestion
- Frequent belching
- Excessive thirst

HOW TO STRETCH

1 Kneel leaning backwards while supporting your weight on the palms of your hands.

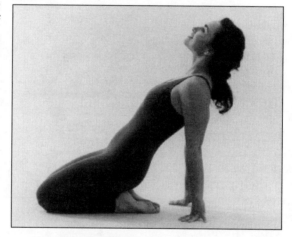

2 Breathe in deeply and slowly as you gently lean backward. Arch your back and lower your head until you feel the tension. Hold this position for a moment, then exhale completely.

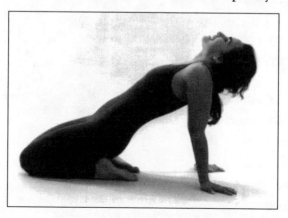

HEART MERIDIAN

THE HEART MERIDIAN and sinew begin at the heart, travel over the chest to the armpit and descend along the underside of your arm past your elbow and wrist to your little finger.

SYMPTOMS OF IMBALANCE

- Pain on the midline of your elbow or arm
- Excessive nervousness
- Insomnia
- Tendency to tire quickly
- Sweaty palms

HOW TO STRETCH

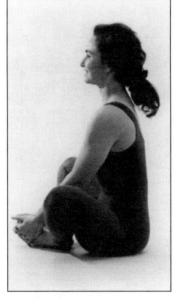

1 Sit on the floor with your spine straight. Hold the toes of both feet with both hands and pull your feet inward so that your knees bend toward the outside of your body.

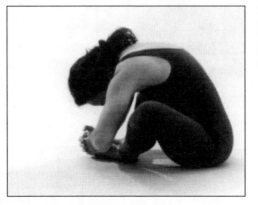

2 Breathe in deeply and slowly as you bend forward over your feet. When you feel the tension, hold the position for a moment, then exhale completely.

SMALL INTESTINE MERIDIAN

THE SMALL INTESTINE meridian and sinew begin at the outer edge of the little finger and travel upward along the side of your hand and across your wrist. The meridian then continues up the back of your arm to your elbow at the midline. From there it runs up your upper arm to the back of your shoulder joint, where it zig-zags around the shoulder blade area and up the back of your neck.

HOW TO STRETCH

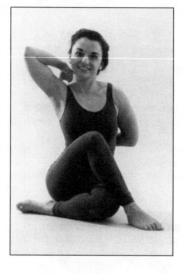

1 Sit with your left leg bent beneath your right leg.

2 Reach over the top of your right shoulder with your right hand while reaching behind your back with your left hand.

SYMPTOMS OF IMBALANCE

- Legs that feel heavy and weak

- Any muscle pain, stiffness, weakness or spasms in your neck

- Pain or stiffness in your shoulders

- Tingling sensations felt downward toward your little finger

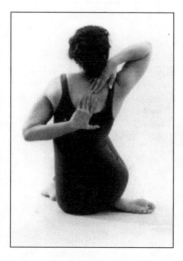

3 As you breathe deeply and slowly, try to touch one hand with the other. When you feel tension, pause for a moment and exhale completely.

4 Reverse your legs and arms, then repeat on your opposite side.

BLADDER MERIDIAN

THE BLADDER MERIDIAN

THE BLADDER MERIDI-AN pathway contains more acupoints than any other. It follows two lines on both sides of the spine. These two paths join on the lower thighs, then descend the back of your legs to your feet. The sinew associated with the bladder meridian forms the groove you use to guide the balls from one point to the next. This sinew includes the muscles located on the back of the buttocks and leg which you activate using the Acupressure Warmup.

The bladder meridian begins at the inside corners of your eyes, crosses the top of your head, divides into two branches at the back of your neck and descends the entire back to the lower thigh. Here the two branches join and follow the back of your legs through the gastrocnemius muscle to the ankles and then to the little toe.

HOW TO STRETCH

SYMPTOMS OF IMBALANCE

- Stiffness, tightness or pain along your spine
- Back spasms
- Sciatica
- Difficulty bending over
- Tight hamstrings
- Tight calf muscles
- Stiffness or pain when tilting your head to look downward
- Headaches located at the back of your head
- Tight Achilles tendon.

1 Sit and pull your knees close to your chest with your toes pointed forward.

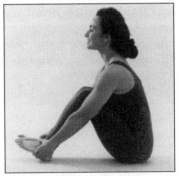

2 Breathe deeply as you slowly push forward, stretching your body over your legs. Pause for a moment, then exhale completely.

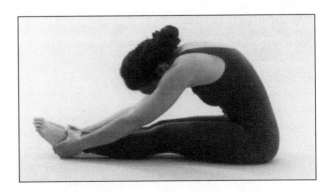

KIDNEY MERIDIAN

THE KIDNEY MERIDIAN starts on the underside of your little toe, then crosses the bottom of your foot at an angle to rise from under the foot beneath the inner ankle. It travels up the back side of your lower leg along the midline, then crosses the gastrocnemius, passes the knee crease at the midline and continues up the leg to link with the spinal column.

HOW TO STRETCH

1 Lie flat on your back on the floor.

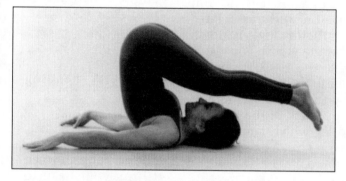

SYMPTOMS OF IMBALANCE

• Weak and brittle bones

• Tension and lack of mobility in the waist area

• Tightness of the stomach muscles

• Cramping on the bottom of the foot

• Extreme fatigue

• Edema

2 Begin inhaling slowly and deeply while you raise both legs and your trunk over your head keeping your knees fairly straight.

3 As you reach the point of tension pause for a moment and exhale completely.

NOTE: When done correctly this is an extremely effective posture. However, when done incorrectly this exercise can damage the muscles along the spine. When doing this stretch take great care not to over-stretch. Go to the point of tension but not beyond. Attempting to push or "bounce" beyond the point of tension could injure your back.

PERICARDIUM MERIDIAN

THE PERICARDIUM meridian begins in the chest and travels across it to the fold of skin at your armpit. It then progresses around the edge of your armpit to descend the middle of your upper arm through the forearm between the tendons that lead to your wrist. From there it crosses your palm into your middle finger.

SYMPTOMS OF IMBALANCE

• Numbness extending into your fingers

• Chest pains

• Heart problems

• Circulatory problems

• Abnormal blood pressure making vigorous exercise impossible

• Nausea

• Vomiting

HOW TO STRETCH

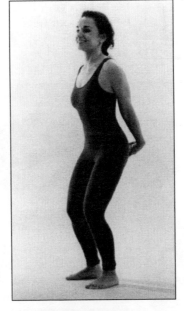

1 Stand with your knees slightly bent and your legs about shoulder width apart. Clasp your hands behind your back.

2 Breathe in deeply and slowly as you raise your arms behind your back while keeping your elbows straight. When you start to feel tension, hold the position for a moment.

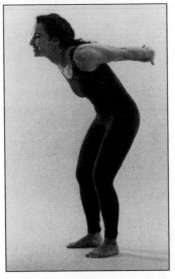

3 Exhale completely while still in the stretch position.

TRIPLE WARMER MERIDIAN

THE TRIPLE WARMER meridian begins on the fourth finger and travels up the backside of your hand between the bones that extend from the fourth and fifth fingers to the wrist. From there it proceeds up the back of your arm on the midline, over the elbow and up the midline of your upper arm. It traverses the top of the shoulder, crosses the neck beneath the ear, circles the ear and ends near the outside corner of the eye.

SYMPTOMS OF IMBALANCE

- Pain or stiffness in the region of the neck and shoulders
- Wrist pain
- Tennis elbow
- Headaches located on the side of the head

HOW TO STRETCH

1 Lie flat on your back with your hands clasped beneath your head.

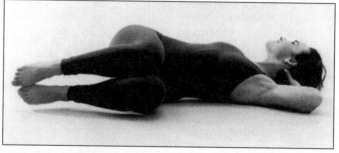

2 Hold your knees together as you breathe in deeply and slowly while rolling your knees to your left. At the end of your exhalation twist from the hip until you feel tension. Hold for a moment, then exhale completely.

3 Relax, then repeat on the opposite side.

GALLBLADDER MERIDIAN

THE GALLBLADDER meridian is long and complex. It begins near the outer corner of the eye and rises to the hairline at the edge of the forehead (in the area where many people's hairlines recede). From there it twice loops from the front to the back of the head before running down the neck, across the back of the shoulders to the location of SI-12, DISAPPEARING TENSION. From there it travels down the front of the shoulders, back and forth across the chest and flanks to arrive at GB-30. From there it proceeds down the center of the outside of the leg, in front of the ankle, over the top of the foot and out to the tip of the little toe.

SYMPTOMS OF IMBALANCE

- Strains and sprains on any outer part of the legs, or knees

- Difficulty bending and straightening the knee

- Pelvic region sprains

- Pain in the hips and flanks

- Pain in the sides of the chest and neck

HOW TO STRETCH

1 Sit with your right leg crossed over your left leg (with your left leg, bent at the knee, underneath).

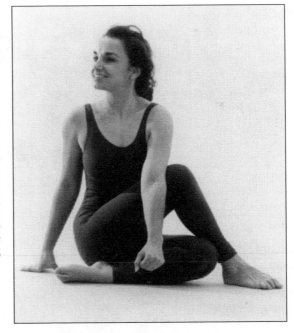

2 Breathe in deeply and slowly as you turn to your right. When you feel the tension, hold the position for a moment, then exhale completely.

3 Switch legs, then repeat on the opposite side.

LIVER MERIDIAN

THE LIVER MERIDIAN stretch is last in the stretching sequence. The liver meridian begins on the top side of the big toe and travels between the big toe and the second toe. It passes the upper, inner ankle and the inside of the leg to the groin. From the groin it angles up the flanks to beneath the ribs, where it crosses to the chest beneath the lung.

HOW TO STRETCH

1 Sit with your hands clasped, extended over your head and your legs bent outward as far as you can without feeling tension.

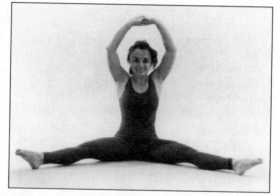

SYMPTOMS OF IMBALANCE

- Weakness in the joints
- Instability of the joints
- General stiffness of the muscles
- Pain on the inner side of the knee and leg
- Pain in the groin area

2 Breathe in deeply and slowly as you bend to the right. Keep your torso parallel to your leg on the side toward which you bend. Stop when you feel tension, hold for a moment and exhale completely.

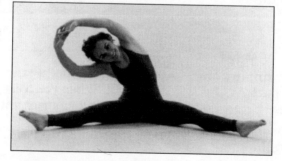

3 Sit straight, relax and repeat process on the opposite side.

FLEXIBILITY TESTS

FLEXIBILITY TESTS

THE TESTS PRESENTED here are used to measure flexibility for the purpose of evaluating sports potential. The measurements you will take will be less accurate than those obtained by experienced testers using professional equipment. However, if you keep your testing conditions relatively similar and chart you progress in a consistent manner, you will be able to judge where you need improvement. In professional application some of these numbers are subtracted from measures of physical stature, such as height, width of shoulders or length of arms. Since you are recording only your own progress, this step is not required. What is important is to establish an easily recorded measure by which you can monitor your overall improvement.

The tests are suitable for anyone capable of performing them, including children as young as seven or eight years old. All of these tests are applicable to both male and female athletes. However, you will need a helper. As you will see in the photographs, your helper can be anyone, even a child. Because the measurements are simple, you will only need two yardsticks and a cloth measuring tape like one used for sewing.

Keep in mind that flexibility is relative. You may be very flexible in one area and less flexible in another. Thus you are not likely to be equally flexible in all of the tests. Please remember to follow the philosophy we have discussed throughout this book — don't force or strain or make yourself uncomfortable. Simply measure the point at which you feel muscular tension. These flexibility tests shouldn't become a competition with yourself or others. They are meant only as an easy way to quantify the improvement you will feel for yourself.

The first time you do the tests, choose a time when you have an hour free. Perform each of these tests before doing the Acupressure Warmup. Record your initial scores. Then, complete the Acupressure Warmup and test yourself again. Not only will you feel a difference; but in many cases you will be able to measure that difference immediately.

After the first month of doing the Acupressure Warmup, do the tests and record your scores again. Compare these new scores to those you recorded the first time. You should see a real difference, depending on your state of fitness when you began. By recording and comparing scores every month or so, you can clearly confirm the improvement you will already feel. When the scores stabilize, you will have reached a higher level of conditioning. You will also have trained yourself so that your sensitivity will be your own best test.

The Acupressure Warmup works whether you record your scores or not. The tests are just an easy way to show yourself your progress. If you are young, or in excellent condition at any age, you will not see dramatic improvement in your flex-test scores. This is because you already have considerable flexibility. If, on the other hand, you are just beginning a fitness program, you will see greater change in your scores.

Even the fittest athlete can benefit from an occasional use of the flex-tests. By keeping track of your progress you will be able to identify where you need more work, where you should concentrate your effort, how best to use your limited time, and how to customize the Warmup for yourself.

Don't push for "better" scores. Use the tests to monitor your progress, to be sure that you are paying attention to all aspects of your condition and to guide your use of time efficiently. There is little sense in comparing scores with your friends. Everyone's body is a little different and you are keeping track of your personal progress, not starting a new competitive sport. Save your competitive spirit for the next game! Some people who are in poor physical condition are quite flexible. Others who may be in great shape have difficulty with some motion.

> ### TOM
>
> *Tom is a physical therapist at the hospital where we conducted our acupressure research. To demonstrate the procedure and to determine the research protocol, we needed a volunteer. Tom, because of his stiff and painful back, was the one we felt would best demonstrate the test.*
>
> *We measured Tom before and after acupressure. His range of motion had increased more than 15% in all of the range of motion tests. Most patients in the study have shown the same level of increased flexibility.*

TRUNK AND NECK EXTENSION

THIS TEST MEASURES the flexibility of your back and neck. This flexibility is required by many movements in sports. While most obviously seen in back-arching activities such as gymnastics, trunk and neck flexibility is often challenged by contact sports such as football and wrestling.

OBJECT

To measure the maximum height above the floor that you can raise your trunk and neck. This measures your ability to hyperextend your trunk.

EQUIPMENT

One yardstick

PERFORMANCE

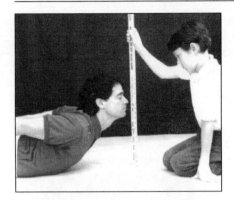

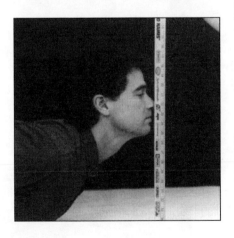

1

Lie face down on the floor with your hands clasped behind your back and your helper sitting directly in front of you.

2

Raise your neck and trunk until the tension makes you want to stop. Your helper will be holding the yardstick vertically next to your nose.

3

Measure the distance from the floor to the tip of your nose.

RECORDING YOUR SCORES

Record the distance from the floor to the tip of your nose.

ANKLE FLEXION TEST

THE ANKLES are often a weak point and are, along with the knees, among the most frequent sites of injury. Any sport that involves running, jumping, quick starts and stops stresses the ankles. Thus ankle flexibility is a performance factor in skiing, biking, horizontal distance jumps, and sprints.

OBJECT

To measure the greatest forward lean (ankle flexion) possible without pain.

EQUIPMENT

One yardstick

PERFORMANCE

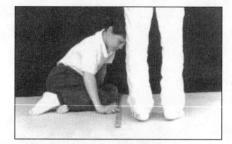

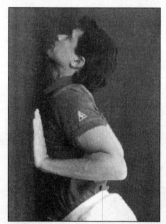

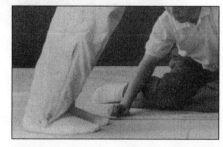

1

Stand with your chest against a wall with your feet about shoulder width apart and your heels flat on the floor. Have your helper position a yardstick so he or she can measure the distance between the wall and your toes.

2

Move progressively away from the wall until you reach the maximum distance from which you can lean forward while keeping your knees straight and your chest, chin and arms flat against the wall. Do not lean so far forward as to cause pain.

3

Have your helper measure the distance between your toe line and the wall.

RECORDING YOUR SCORES

Record the distance from the wall to your toe line.
NOTE: It takes a little practice to get the distance right. If you stand too close to the wall, the flexion will be insufficient. If you stand too far back, you won't be able to keep your heels flat on the floor without forcing your muscles. If you move too far backward and you feel excess tension or pain while leaning forward, push away with your arms and reposition your feet.

SHOULDER ROTATION

PERFORMANCE

THIS TEST MEASURES the range of rotation motion possible for your shoulders. This motion is easily seen in the back stroke in swimming and the ring events in gymnastics. However, shoulder rotation also plays an important role in tennis, golf and baseball, sports where swinging motions are critical to good performance.

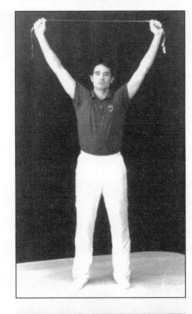

1

Stand with your feet shoulder width apart grasping the midpoint of the tape measure with the thumb and index finger of both hands. Raise your arms in front, keeping your elbows straight.

2

Raise both arms above your head letting the tape measure slide through your fingers only as much as is necessary to rotate your arms.

OBJECT

To measure your ability to rotate your shoulders with as little distance between the arms and hands as possible.

EQUIPMENT

Flexible tape measure

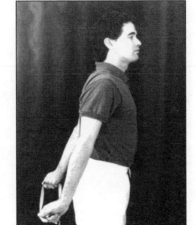

3

Continue to rotate your shoulders, keeping your elbows straight, until you complete the rotation.

RECORDING YOUR SCORES

Upon completion of this rotation, measure the distance between the grip points on the tape measure. A smaller distance indicates greater flexibility.

BRIDGE UP

THIS TEST MEASURES spinal flexibility. A flexible spine is important for any movement skill but it is critical for athletic events like the butterfly stroke in swimming, gymnastics, modern dance, or ballet. This test is difficult for some. If this is true for you, your helper must take the measurement quickly. Position your thumbs next to your ears before you make the upward push. Don't force yourself; if you have difficulty pushing far enough upward to lift your head from the floor, just measure the maximum arch possible without lifting your head.

OBJECT

To measure the distance between the floor and the highest point of the arch in your back. This measures the hyperextension of your spine.

EQUIPMENT

Two yardsticks

PERFORMANCE

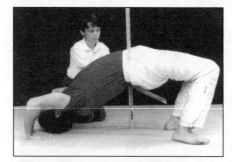

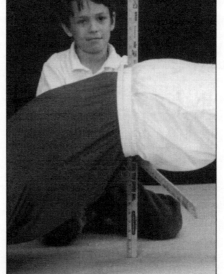

1

Lie flat on the floor with your arms and legs bent, soles down.

2

Walk your hands and feet closer together as your helper crosses the yardsticks at a 90 degree angle and slides the horizontal yardstick beneath the arch of your back.

3

Arch your back until the tension you feel makes you want to stop. Your helper must measure the distance between the high point of your back and the floor.

RECORDING YOUR SCORES

Record the distance between the highest point of the arch of your back and the floor.

SIT AND REACH

THIS IS A VERY RELIABLE test. It was selected because people with low-back problems often have restricted flexibility in the hamstring muscles and lower back. This forward-bending motion is critical in many sports: vaulting, diving, trampoline, track and field, basketball, tennis, and gymnastics. It is important in almost all physical activities, even your household chores.

OBJECT

To measure how far your finger tips can be extended beyond the line formed by your heels when your legs are fully extended. This measures the flexion of your hip and your back and the suppleness of your hamstrings.

EQUIPMENT

Two Yardsticks

PERFORMANCE

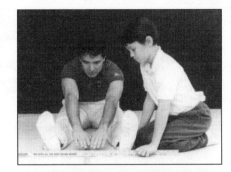

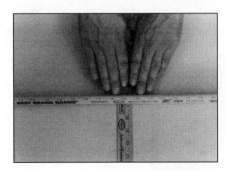

1
Remove your footgear and sit on the floor with your legs fully extended (knees flat on the floor).

2
Position the first yardstick so that it is parallel to your legs, centered between your legs, and its midpoint (18 inch mark) even with your heels. Cross the second yardstick at 90 degrees, at a point even with the edge of your heels.

3
Reach forward until the tension in your muscles stops you.

4
Have your helper move the crossing yardstick forward to mark the farthest point reached by your finger tips.

RECORDING YOUR SCORES

Measure the distance from the line of your heels that you were able to reach without pain. Some people cannot reach their heels. If this is the case record the distance to the midpoint, for example, "-2" meaning two inches short of the heels.

SHOULDER AND WRIST

THIS EXERCISE TESTS the ability of your shoulders and wrist to flex backward. This flexibility is employed in throwing motions of every kind, and in many swings, even those with a side-arm motion.

OBJECT

To measure your ability to raise your shoulders.

EQUIPMENT

Two yardsticks

PERFORMANCE

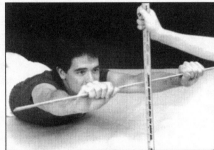

1

Lie face down on the floor with your arms extended in front of you about shoulder width apart. Grasp one yardstick in both hands. Your helper sits directly in front of you holding the vertical yardstick.

2

Keep your elbows straight and lift the yardstick as high as you can before the tension becomes pain.

3

Measure the maximum height reached on the vertical yardstick.

RECORDING YOUR SCORES

Record the distance from the floor to the maximum height reached.

NOTE: Some people are so flexible that they can reach well above the line of their back. Record the highest score. If you are this flexible, it is not likely that you will show large improvements over time; however, the measurement is still a valid baseline for your individual condition.

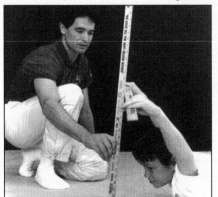

REFERENCE SECTION

HISTORY OF ACUPRESSURE

ACUPRESSURE IS PART of an ancient Oriental medical system that is surprisingly similar to our most modern ideas of health. We have learned that our daily attitudes and activities influence our well-being. We sometimes call this idea "holism," or simply talk about a "healthy lifestyle." Very early in their history the Chinese recognized the same relationship. They used the idea of "qi" (pronounced "chee") to explain how internal and external influences affected their lives.

Chinese physicians thought in terms of many qi: influences from the weather, the environment, people, places, activities, and work. For example, the Chinese observed that a cold-damp environment was harmful. Thus, they referred to "cold-damp qi" as a pathogen, a cause of disease. Today, we might say that the cold and damp environment produced the physical causes of disease by, for example, making it difficult for us to maintain body temperature. Whether we call the problem "cold-damp qi" or "a thermoregulation disorder," the relationship is the same: prolonged exposure to cold and damp can lead to dull pain, heaviness and numbness in the joints and limbs. Disease and disability were thought of as disturbances in a balance of qualities that was health.

Thus, Chinese medicine combined diet, natural drugs, massage, movement exercise, and acupuncture into a sophisticated health care system. When we experience tight, tense muscles we are experiencing what Chinese doctors called "qi stagnation." Several of the Acupressure Warmup points ensure freely flowing qi and were thought of by the Chinese as "disinhibiting," restoring the free flow of qi. Bruises are a "blood and qi accumulation," and the solution is to move the blood and qi. Some Acupressure Warmup points have this purpose. In short, the Acupressure Warmup points, all of which have been known to Oriental doctors for centuries, activate processes in the human body which benefit the conditions that athletes commonly experience.

How Old is Acupressure?

NO ONE REALLY KNOWS when acupressure began, where it first developed, or exactly how it was discovered. It is very likely that acupressure developed first and that acupuncture followed as ancient Chinese physicians gained greater knowledge. It is a practice so honored in the East that legend credits its discovery to the cultural heroes who are symbolic of the development of agriculture, science, government and religion in Asian culture. Its most important ideas are basic to Eastern civilization. Earlier in this century, Chinese writers believed acupuncture to be 5,000 years old. While that date is doubtful, it is clear that acupuncture is part of the world's oldest continuously-used medical system.

Recent archeological discoveries include technical manuscripts describing the acupuncture meridians and points. These are reliably dated to about 200 B.C. When Marco Polo arrived in China he was impressed that acupuncture cured diseases that were feared in Europe. We also know that by the seventeenth century the Chinese had made many of the discoveries that were to revolutionize medicine in the West. They understood blood circulation, anatomical relationships, and even used an early version of vaccination against smallpox. Acupuncture's influence on the West was very gradual. When the Portuguese navigators arrived in the Far East, they recorded acupuncture for export to Europe. The books they wrote still exist. Yet, it wasn't until this century that acupuncture had a significant influence on the West.

For forty years beginning in 1900 the first modern scholar to study acupuncture, Georges Soulie De Morant, worked and studied side by side with the best Chinese physicians. Although his work did not receive the Nobel Prize for which it was nominated, it did introduce acupuncture to French physicians. Ironically, the ensuing spread of acupressure and acupuncture through Europe did not influence many people in the U.S. James Reston, a journalist accompanying Richard Nixon to China, experienced emergency surgery using acupuncture anesthesia. It was his reports that awoke interest here.

If you find the history of acupuncture as fascinating as I do, there is a reading list at the end of the book. However, what is most important to us today is that both ancient and modern Chinese doctors have done what good physicians do everywhere — kept careful records of their experience and results. It is from this legacy of practical experience that the Acupressure Warmup evolved.

How Does Acupressure Work?

Even among the best scientific minds there is no absolute agreement on the mechanisms by which acupuncture or acupressure work. Serious study has only recently begun. However, as scientists have been able to measure ever more subtle chemical and electrical signals in the body, our image of human function has changed. At the leading edge of science, the human body is no longer seen as a collection of complex mechanical devices. Rather, it is thought to be more like a vastly flexible computer. Thousands and thousands of signals, some chemical, some electrical, carry millions and millions of messages that govern how everything works. In this advanced view we can see that heat and pressure are natural signals that could influence the body's controlling network.

From studies done by Western scientists we know that the acupuncture meridians and points can be traced and measured electrically. Scientists have also shown that acupuncture produces higher levels of important biochemicals. We know that it increases the availability of substances that play important roles in the control of pain. Other studies show that gentle stimulation can increase flows in even the deepest body tissues. Some scientists have shown that the electrically active fascia, the tissues that wrap and interconnect the whole body, could be the location of a sensitive communications network.

In brief, we now know that very tiny signals are produced by, and can influence, even individual cells. Thus, the application of heat or pressure can cause many responses. Nerves can be stimulated, tiny electrical signals generated, and the minute electrical and magnetic fields that surround each cell can be changed. The changes can, in turn, inform the body's many regulatory processes that it is time to start, stop, work harder, or respond in some way.

From the work of scientists we can imagine that the meridians and points are like the strings and frets of a guitar. Pressing each string at each different position produces a different note. Like a musical score, the Acupressure Warmup lets us do more than produce sounds at random. Just as a guitarist will choose notes that are melodious, we can select a combination of points that balance our condition. When we activate these points our bodies will begin to function more harmoniously. When the Acupressure Warmup points are activated, they signal body functions to start or stop, flow more or less, modify or change. In short, they send messages that influence our wellbeing.

In a way, we can think of the Acupressure Warmup as the overture to the complex body symphony of sports. The Acupressure Warmup takes advantage of the fact that pressure alone safely provides many of the benefits of acupuncture. Using a simple technique, the Acupressure Warmup produces physiological changes that benefit the anatomical areas and functions that we stress in sports. Regardless of how it works, the Acupressure Warmup is a practical blend of professional clinical experience, and the feedback of both professional and amateur athletes.

READER'S GUIDE

Oriental Exercise Systems

The Essential Movements of Tai Chi, by John Kotsias, Paradigm Publications, Brookline, MA, 1989.

This is a step by step guide to the basic movements of the Oriental martial arts — tai chi and qi gong, the "qi cultivation" exercises. It includes many diagrams and is arranged for self-teaching.

Zen Imagery Exercises, by Shizuto Masunaga, Japan Publications, Tokyo, 1987.

This book provides a full set of instructions for many meridian exercises. It is arranged for self-teaching with many photographs and drawings and has discussions of breathing, relaxation and imagery in movement.

Oriental History and Culture

The Layman's Guide to Acupuncture, by Yoshio Manaka, John Weatherhill Inc., New York, NY, 1972.

This is a basic introduction to acupuncture by one of the most important researchers of the modern era. It is easily read by laypersons but has some information for those with a particular interest in medicine and science.

Medicine in China: A History of Ideas, by Paul U. Unschuld, University of California Press, Berkeley CA, 1983.

Paul Unschuld, one of the leading authorities on Chinese medicine, presents a solid intellectual history in this text. The book is fascinating and can be enjoyed without a specialized background. However, it is not a casual text and is best for readers who have a more-than-casual interest.

Technical Information About Acupoints and Meridians

The Fundamentals of Chinese Acupuncture, by Andrew Ellis, Nigel Wiseman and Ken Boss, Paradigm Publications, Brookline, MA, 1988.

This book is actually an advanced professional text used in physician education programs. Although this book contains much information that will not be of interest to the layperson, it is a good choice for lay readers because compared to most "point books" it is relatively inexpensive and includes many more illustrations.

BIBLIOGRAPHY

Becker, R.O. and G. Selden, *The Body Electric*, New York: William Morrow, 1985.

Ellis, A., N. Wiseman and K. Boss, *Fundamentals of Chinese Acupuncture*, Brookline, MA: Paradigm Publications, 1988.

Ellis, A., N. Wiseman and K. Boss, *Grasping the Wind,* Brookline, MA: Paradigm Publications, 1989.

Hashimoto, K. and Y. Kawakami, *Sotai: Balance and Health Through Natural Movement*, Tokyo: Japan Publications, 1983.

Manaka, Y., K. Itaya and S.Birch, *Chasing the Dragon's Tail*, Brookline, MA: Paradigm Publications, 1992.

Matsumoto, K. and S. Birch, *Hara Diagnosis: Reflections on the Sea*, Brookline, MA: Paradigm Publications, 1988.

Needham, J and Lu Gwei-Djen, *Celestial Lancets: A History and Rationale of Acupuncture and Moxibustion*, Cambridge, England: Cambridge University Press, 1980.

Needham, J., *Science and Civilization in China, volume 2*, Cambridge, England: Cambridge University Press, 1956.

Unschuld, P., *Medicine in China: A History of Ideas*, Berkeley, CA: University of California Press, 1983.

Unschuld, P., *Medicine in China: Nan Ching, the Classic of Difficult Issues*, Berkeley, CA: University of California Press, 1986.

INDEX

126

INDEX

INDEX

ankle: 100; inner side of knee: 100, 108; inner side of leg: 108; inner side of lower leg: 100; jaw: 99; mid back region: 100; middle of back: 99; midline of arm: 101; midline of elbow: 101; neck and shoulder region: 106; neck muscles: 102; of muscles: throughout body: 74; recurring: 7; shoulder: 18, 102; sides of chest and neck: 107; when doing push ups: 97; when tilting head to look down: 103; when turning head: 98; wrist: 106

palms, sweaty: 101

patella: 71

pelvic bone: 44

pelvic girdle: 54

pelvic region, muscular imbalance: 46; sprains: 107

pelvis: 54; anterior tilt: 42; slight rotation of: 84; upper: 47

perception, diminished field of: 10

physical condition, poor: 112

posture, slumping: 30

PUSHING AWAY: 18, 26, 80-81

Q

qi: 121; cold-damp: 121; stagnation: 121

qi gong: 5, 96, 124

R

racquet sports: 18; backhand motion painful or hard: 18; injuries in: 22

range of movement, reduced: 3

respiratory limitations: 80

respiratory problems: 26, 80, 97

ROW THE BOAT: 10, 30-33

rowing exercises: 18

running, limited fluidity: 46

S

sacral hiatus: 51

sacrum: 47-48

scapula: 32, 33, 35-36

scar tissue: 3

sciatica: 50, 57, 103

SCISSORS KICK: 70, 84-85

shin splints: 86, 99

shoulder blades, pain or stiffness between: 97

SHOULDER MOUNTAIN: 18, 22 -25

SHOULDER VALLEY: 18-21

shoulders, forward rotation of: 80; hunched: 26, 97; limited range of motion: 22; pain or stiffness of: 102, 106; range of motion of: 115; tension in: 99

SI-10: 18-21

SI-12: 10, 14-17, 21

SIDE TO SIDE: 50, 62-65

sinew: 94, 95

sit ups, difficulty doing: 99

spasms, back: 103; neck muscles: 102

spine, stiff, tight, painful along: 103

sprain, outer part of leg or knee: 107; pain and stiffness of: 86; sprain, pelvic region: 107

SPRINTER'S VALLEY: 54, 58-62

ST-31: 50, 66-70, 72

ST-32: 62, 68, 70-73

stair climbing: 46

stamina, lack of: 97

STEPPING UP: 34, 38, 46-50

stiffness: 3; along spine: 103; back: 112; between shoulder blades: 97; inner side of ankle: 100; inner side of knee: 100; inner side of lower leg: 100; mid back region: 100; neck and shoulder region: 106; neck muscles: 102; of muscles: 108; shoulders: 102; when tilting head to look down: 103; when turning head: 98

stomach muscles, tightness of: 104

strain: 6; constant on back: 46; outer part of leg or knee: 107

strains, of muscles: throughout body: 74

strength, lack of physical: 98; of entire muscular system: 86

stress: 38; neck: 10; on lower back: 46; upper back: 10

stretching: 3-4, 96

surgery, due to injury: 3

T

tai chi: 5, 96, 124

tail bone: 48, 51

tennis elbow: 82, 98, 106

tension: 14; in shoulders: 99; middle of back: 99; waist area: 104; when raising arms in front of body: 26

thermoregulation disorder: 121

thigh: 55; strength and flexibility of: 84

THIGH GATE: 50, 66-70, 72

thirst, excessive: 100

throwing motion: 18; difficulties of: 22

tightness, along spine: 103; shoulder: 18 stomach muscles: 104

tingling sensations, downward to little finger: 102

tiring, quickly: 101

trunk and neck, flexibility of: 113

TWISTING AROUND: 34-38

U

upper body, rotation: 34

UPPER BODY SUPPORT: 46, 54-57

V

vein, cephalic: 80; small saphenous: 88

vomiting: 105

W

waist, tension and lack of mobility: 104

walking, limited fluidity: 46

weakness, joints: 108; neck muscles: 102; when doing push ups: 97

wheezing: 26

wrist inflexibility: 99

wrist pain: 106

Y

yoga postures: 93